YO-DKN-003

A Word From the Editors

We love our children. We want them to be safe, healthy, and happy. We want to provide the best opportunities for them to grow in faith and in knowledge to become adults committed to God through Jesus Christ. We want them to grow up and have satisfying lives and vocations. We want our children to grow up.

➤ AIDS kills adults, teenagers, and children.
➤ AIDS infects the poor, the middle class, the wealthy, the educated, and the uneducated.
➤ AIDS is most often spread by sexual activity and injection drug use. It is also spread by ignorance, apathy, and denial.
➤ AIDS is in the church, and it is a controversial and uncomfortable topic.

Education Is the Best Defense

There is no question in or outside of the church that AIDS is a devastating disease and that one way or another, it is having a profound affect on all of us. But AIDS is a preventable disease, and education is a powerful weapon in this current war against HIV.

The writers in this issue all address head-on the hard facts about AIDS and HIV infection. I expect that the articles and programs will elicit a variety of conflicting emotions and responses from you. What we want for our children and teenagers seems directly counter to what we must consider when we broach the at-risk behaviors that are most typical to HIV infection.

But we must consider those behaviors, because people of all ages and stations in life are becoming infected and dying. The more we know about good choices and intelligent behavior, the better off we all are in the battle against a deadly, but preventable disease. We can't put our heads in the sand and hope AIDS will go away. We have to know what we're dealing with and how to confront it.

The Church's Stance

As in all issues, not every denomination or religious body agrees with other religious groups on their stated positions on HIV/AIDS. But most denominations in the United States have taken stances that are remarkably similar and encouragingly grace-ful. While individual members or groups of members of good conscience within these Protestant and Roman Catholic bodies may disagree, the church, as the agent of God's kingdom on earth, has spoken and strives to uphold a faithful ministry to persons with HIV/AIDS.

Most denominations and religious bodies suggest these points of common need and endeavor:

➤ *The need for education*

Accurate, factual, straightforward, and sensitive sex education is a must, not only for children and youth, but for adults as well. The church is in an advantageous position to include positive moral, ethical, and spiritual guidance in a context that may be lacking or not be permitted in secular or social arenas.

➤ *The sanctity of marriage*

Marriage as a covenant relationship between a man and a woman is the means by which persons live out their intimate, long-term loving, and supportive commitments to each other.

➤ *The goodness of our sexuality*

Sexuality is one of our many gifts from God and we affirm its goodness. Sexual relations are to be expressed within the context of marriage.

➤ *The innate worth of all individuals*

All persons are considered as created in the image of God. Some persons engage in practices that are considered by others to be incompatible with Christian teaching, but that does not exclude them from the bounds of God's grace or from the fellowship of the church.

➤ *The responsible stewardship of our bodies*

The use and/or abuse of alcohol and drugs continues to threaten the physical, emotional, and spiritual well-being of not only the user/abuser, but his or her family as well. Abstinence is the most sure way to defeat the life-threatening effects of these substances. Education about them and their effects should be encouraged.

➤ *The disease as illness, not punishment*

The Gospel challenges all persons to think and act with compassion for those who are ill, not to judge or diagnose the reasons for the disease along with the disease itself. The Bible is clear about God's intent that all persons should be whole in body and in spirit, including persons infected with HIV/AIDS.

The Other Side

Data from responsible and respectable sources such as the Search Institute, as well as our own observations and experience, tell us that not all persons live in ways that totally support the stance of the church. Some teens do engage in sexual activity; some do use illegal intravenous drugs. Not all those teens are outside the church. We cannot truthfully say "Not my kids." Both churched and unchurched youth engage in at-risk behaviors that may infect them with HIV, and that ultimately leads to AIDS.

To the Point: AIDS wholeheartedly supports the stance of the church, but it also supports the need for all teenagers to know what causes AIDS, what doesn't cause AIDS, and how not to become infected. To do that, we talk about sex and drugs. In so doing, we believe we are affirming, and being affirmed by, the Gospel of Jesus Christ, who came that we may have abundant life.

Diana L. Hynson
Carmen M. Gaud
Gail G. Bock

How to Use
To the Point: AIDS

AIDS is a crucial subject for teens today. As an adult worker with youth, you may have found yourself hearing conversations around the fringes of other youth group activities and conversations. You may be looking for program materials that go beyond "Just say no." You realize that there are numerous resources on the market and need to find a choice that allows you a variety of approaches to the subject. You know you need to be able to talk to teens from a biblical and theological context too. "Health 101" is just not enough. This issue of *To the Point* will provide all that and more.

To the Point: AIDS Helps You Help Others

Perhaps one of the most poignant and difficult tasks for you as an adult friend to teens is how to help them when they are hurting, frightened, confused, or angry. The section "When Someone Comes to You" will help you get a handle on how to prepare yourself to confront a difficult subject, and then how to help others from a perspective of care and concern. This segment will provide biblical and theological insights for how we understand and talk about God, death, dying, grace, responsibility, and compassion. Though this is not the first section in the resource, you should consider reading this section first.

To the Point: AIDS Seizes "Teachable Moments"

Not every encounter with the subject of AIDS requires a full program on AIDS or a related topic. But you still want to address that casual question or the pop in visit by several teens to your office at church or the encounter in the hallway.

The first section, "Teaching Articles," provides lots of up-to-date information about AIDS and related issues, like saying no, what every teen needs to know, how some other teens coped with their own AIDS-related situation, what can happen when drugs are around, and more.

You can read these articles for your own information and pass them along. If you're looking for the scoop on AIDS, it's there. If you want to do some intentional activities or begin a profitable discussion, the helps are right there, either on the same or the next page. Mine these articles for ammunition on how to be ready for the teachable moments that teens will offer you. The articles and reflection sections are also suitable for a more formal setting, such as a youth group meeting, sharing group gathering, or other study setting.

We encourage you to pay special attention to the personal stories. Each provides a different slant, or set of values, or cluster of circumstances that will give teens multiple ways to reflect on their own values, behavior, and situations.

To the Point: AIDS Offers Ready-Made Programs

If you want to offer a program or series of programs in the youth fellowship setting, in a retreat, or other organized class, the sections on "Programs" and "More Program Ideas" are the places to begin. The programs give you about forty minutes of discussion, activities, games, and other options for an organized learning setting. The teaching articles can easily be adapted for formal settings as well. And the program ideas offer added helps for how to begin and sustain a discussion and other hints.

To the Point: AIDS Gives You Leader's Guides

Spread the Word: Teens Talk to Teens About AIDS is a video available from EcuFilm and also from Cokesbury. The video comes with its own leader's guide, but that guide doesn't deal with any biblical or theological approaches to AIDS. The guide in *To the Point: AIDS* does. Now when you rent or buy the video, you have two options for leading discussion and for delving into the wealth of ideas and insights from the video: the EcuFilm guide and the guide provided here.

The video is about 30 minutes long and can be used in an organized setting, with another program or retreat, or for individual viewing.

The other leader's guide is for Magic Johnson's book, *What You Can Do to Avoid AIDS*. This guide provides questions and comments as discussion starters for each chapter.

To the Point: AIDS Has Solid Support Materials

Included are sections for worship resources, basic facts and information, where to go for help, and what other print resources are available. Much of this information is printed in English and in Spanish.

To the Point: AIDS tiene un sección en Español

Vea la sección en las paginas 65-82.

Incluye programas, ideas para la enseñanza, oraciones y recursos litúrgicos. Contiene un artículo con sugerencias sobre cómo aprovechar mejor este recurso.

Teaching Articles

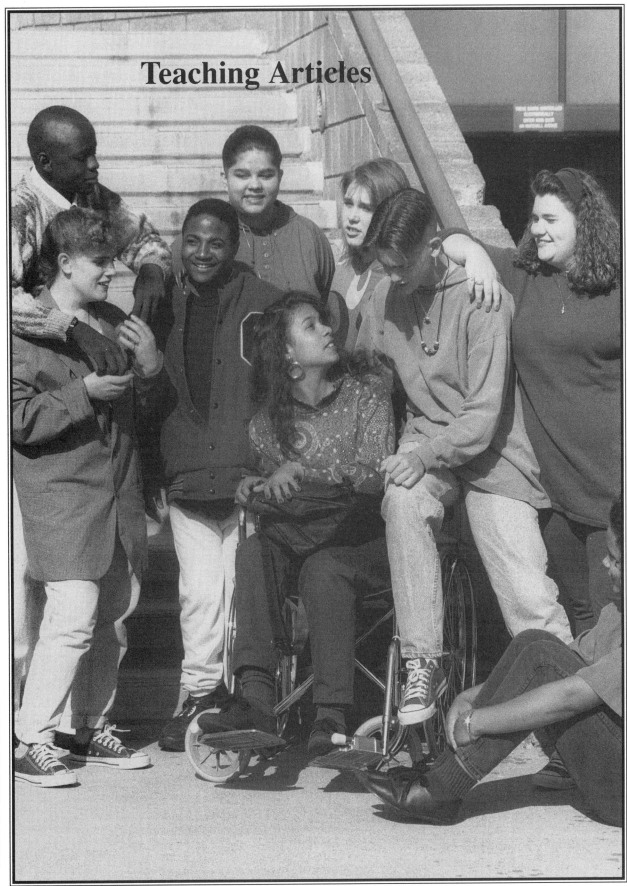

UPDATE: Teens and HIV/AIDS

"What do teenagers really need to know about AIDS?" That's the question I asked a number of teenagers I know. Without exception they told me:

➤ How you can catch AIDS.
➤ How you don't get AIDS (What are the myths?).
➤ How to keep safe from catching AIDS.

I hope you can use this information to protect yourself and the people you care about from exposure to AIDS.

How You Can Catch AIDS

First of all, you can get AIDS because of what you do and not because of who you are. You can catch or give someone HIV (the virus that causes AIDS) if you participate in certain behaviors. HIV is a virus that does not discriminate. AIDS does not care what our skin color or age is, and it doesn't care whether we are male or female. Some people will say: "You can only get AIDS if you are a gay man" or "You can only get AIDS if you shoot drugs!" Wrong. There are lots of people who have gotten AIDS who are not drug users or gay.

The main ways that most teens will be exposed to the AIDS virus is through the high risk behaviors of unprotected sexual contact and intravenous (IV) drug use.

Sexual contact is any contact between a person's genitals (sexual organs) and another person's genitals, mouth, or anus. This means there are a number of sexual activities that can spread the AIDS virus: vaginal sex, oral sex, or anal sex. In any of these activities there is the possibility for the AIDS virus to be spread through bodily fluids (blood, semen, and vaginal secretions) to the mucous membranes (moist linings of the openings to your body). Every time you have unprotected sexual intercourse with another person, male or female, you are exposed to every illness to which that person and his or her previous sexual partners have been exposed.

Unprotected sexual contact is a very risky activity. Young women should especially keep in mind that many young men don't like to admit to bisexual activity. Some guys will have sex with another man and not talk about it with anyone. Then having unprotected sex with that guy can expose a girl to the AIDS virus.

Intravenous drug use is another way that teens can be exposed to HIV. Some people shoot drugs into their veins to get high. Others will do it to pump up on steroids. Either way, IV drug use can be dangerous to your body, causing permanent damage to your internal organs. When people share the same needles ("works") for drugs or steroids, the tiny amounts of blood left in the needle will spread the AIDS virus.

You can also spread AIDS by sharing needles to pierce your ears or make tattoos. Always go to a professional who uses sterile equipment for piercing and tattooing.

If a woman has AIDS or HIV, she can transmit the virus to her unborn child either in the womb or during the birth of the baby. An infected mother can also pass the disease to her child while breast-feeding.

Before 1985 when a test was developed to detect the AIDS virus in blood, some people were infected through blood transfusions. This included many hemophiliacs, who often need donated blood because their own blood does not clot. Today our nation's blood supply is much safer because every unit of donated blood is tested for HIV. People who participate in high risk behaviors are discouraged from donating blood. A small number of health-care workers have been infected with the AIDS virus during accidents, such as being stuck by a needle while drawing blood from an infected patient.

Some people like to blame a person for catching a disease like AIDS by saying: "It's God's will; God is punishing you for sin." Our God is a loving God who does not punish people with diseases. Diseases may teach us lessons about activities that are not good for us—but God is not using diseases to punish us. People who tell you this are using God as a weapon to control you rather than offering you the love that God showed us through Jesus. In **Romans 8:31-39**, Paul reminds us there is nothing in all creation that can ever separate us from the love of God, which is ours through Christ Jesus our Lord.

How Not to Catch AIDS

AIDS is an infectious disease, but it is not like a common cold, which you can catch by breathing the same air or touching a person. You cannot get AIDS from being in the same room with a person with AIDS. You cannot get AIDS by sharing a locker with someone or by drinking from a water fountain after someone with the virus. You cannot get AIDS by using the same bathroom or swimming in the same pool with someone with AIDS.

You cannot give or catch AIDS by touching, hugging, shaking or holding hands, or kissing. Experts who have studied AIDS have never found it to be spread by kissing, even though very small amounts of the virus are present in saliva. But remember—you can pass "mono" (infectious mononucleosis) by sharing drinks with your friends or by deep kissing.

You cannot catch AIDS by donating blood at a Red Cross blood drive or hospital. These blood collection groups use only sterile equipment that no one else has used. You cannot get AIDS or HIV by learning and reading about them. Education, being AIDS-smart, is the best way to prevent exposure to AIDS and other sexually transmitted diseases (STDs). You will not catch AIDS by helping someone with AIDS or HIV as part of a ministry group in your church or community.

In biblical times there was a skin disease called leprosy that people were afraid of because they thought you could catch it by touching a leper. People made lepers leave the town and were afraid to get near them. Jesus showed he cared for the lepers and touched them as a way to show God's love and healing for them (**Matthew 8:1-4**).

People with AIDS need your support and friendship. You may be in a class or church with someone with AIDS who needs your friendship. If you are afraid to touch them then maybe you should think of other ways you can be helpful—like running errands, collecting food, or participating in a walk-a-thon. Don't let your fear keep you from sharing God's love with them just because they are sick.

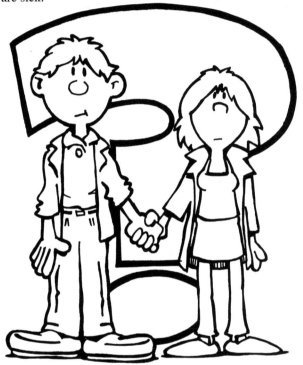

How to Be Safe!

Sex is a special gift from God that we can share in many ways. As boys and girls, teenagers, men and women, sexuality affects who we are and how we interact. There are lots of ways that people interact sexually—from romantic talking, holding hands, kissing, and petting to the very intimate acts involving genital contact.

You should *never* let anyone force you to do anything sexually that makes you uncomfortable or afraid. Your discomfort and fear are signals that you are not ready yet and you are being manipulated or abused by the other person.

Sexual intercourse is one expression of love that should be saved for the person with whom you choose to be in a faithful, monogamous, committed marriage. I know that sounds rough when it seems like a lot of kids are "doing it." But doing it doesn't make them smarter or cooler.

The result of unprotected sexual intercourse can be a baby—and that would change your present and future lifestyle. Or the result can be an STD such as AIDS. The only 100 percent sure way to not expose yourself to AIDS is to not have intimate sexual contact (vaginal, oral, or anal) with anyone. Abstinence from sexual intercourse is the only 100 percent safe alternative and the one your church encourages. There are lots of ways to enjoy your relationships without going all the way.

Persons who have sexual intercourse (vaginal, anal, or oral) should protect both themselves and their partner with a latex condom. A condom (rubber) is an expansive cover for the penis that catches semen when the man ejaculates. Some schools and clinics give condoms to the students. They can also be purchased at all pharmacies and some grocery stores.

Condoms are not 100 percent guaranteed. Sometimes they break or leak. Persons should learn how to use a condom correctly before using it in sexual activity. Persons who use a condom for protection during sexual intercourse should only use a water-based lubricant with nonoxynl-9 (a spermicide that also kills the AIDS virus). A petroleum-based lubricant (baby oil or Vaseline) should never be used on or in a condom—it can weaken the condom or cause it to break. Sexually active persons should care enough about themselves and their partner to share simple protection if they are going to be intimate.

Think about your choices when it comes to sexual activity before you are in a difficult situation where you are forced to do something you aren't ready to do.

The Numbers Can Scare You

If it scares you to know that a lot of teens and young adults who look perfectly healthy are walking around infected with HIV, then you should be scared. The fastest growing portion of the AIDS cases are now among adolescents and young adults. Right now, 20 percent of all new cases of AIDS are for people between the ages of 20 and 29. And since someone can be infected with HIV for five to ten years before it shows up as AIDS, a little simple subtraction will tell you that many young people are being infected while they are teenagers.

Since AIDS was first discovered in 1981 there have been over 242,000 cases reported to the Centers for Disease Control in Atlanta (CDC), and 140,000 of those people have died. More than twice as many people have died from AIDS in the United States as were killed fighting for the United States during the Vietnam War.[1]

But didn't I say that the two ways that teens are catching AIDS/HIV today are by IV drug abuse and sexual activity? The sure solution is clear: Play safe or don't play at all!

———
[1]CDC data as of May 25, 1992.

STD; AIDS; HIV; AZT; CDC— What do all these letters mean?

STD: Sexually Transmitted Disease—an STD is an illness that you can catch or give during intimate sexual activity. These diseases are usually transmitted in sexual intercourse (oral, anal, and vaginal) when bodily fluids (blood, semen, cum, saliva, and vaginal secretions) come in contact with mucous membranes (the wet surfaces of the openings in our bodies). STD's include syphilis, gonorrhea, herpes, genital warts, hepatitis, and AIDS.

AIDS: Acquired Immunodeficiency Syndrome—A disease caused by the HIV, which interferes with your body's natural immune system. AIDS is communicable primarily through sexual activity and unclean IV needle use. Infected women can also pass on the disease to their unborn or nursing children. There is no vaccine to protect you from AIDS or HIV, and there is no cure once you are infected.

HIV: Human Immunodeficiency Virus—the virus (kind of germ or disease-causing agent) that causes AIDS. The only way to tell if you have been exposed to AIDS is a blood test to see if your body is producing antibodies (disease-fighting agents) for HIV. If you have been exposed to HIV, the antibodies may not show up in a test for three to six months. **If you think you have been exposed to HIV, it is important to be tested so you can receive early treatment with drugs that can protect you from some AIDS related diseases.**

AZT: Azidothymidine or Zidovudine—a drug that slows the progress of the disease caused by HIV, allowing infected persons to stay healthy longer.

CDC: Centers for Disease Control—located in Atlanta, GA, keeps up with all the latest information on prevention, control, and treatment of HIV/AIDS and other diseases in the United States.

Chip Aldridge, an ordained United Methodist minister in Alexandria, Virginia, is a member of the AIDS/HIV Committee for the Baltimore-Washington Annual Conference. He is Director of Seminary Relations for Wesley Theological Seminary in Washington, D.C.

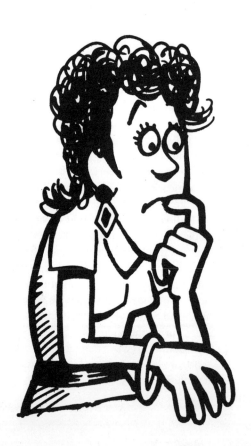

For Further Reflection on "Update: Teens and HIV/AIDS"

A. HIV/AIDS Inventory

Review the substance of this article by taking this inventory of HIV/AIDS information to see how much you already know. Answers are in the article and briefly on page 8.

TRUE OR FALSE:

1 You get HIV/AIDS because of who you are.
2 HIV/AIDS is highly contagious like measles, for example.
3 Babies can be infected with HIV.
4 You get HIV/AIDS from donating blood.
5 Married people can't get HIV/AIDS.
6 HIV/AIDS is a gay disease only.
7 HIV is transmitted by touching, kissing, perspiration, or sneezing.
8 You can become infected with HIV by using intravenous drugs.
9 HIV/AIDS is God's punishment for wrong behavior.
10 There is a cure for HIV/AIDS.
11 Unprotected sex (not using a latex condom and spermicide) is one way to contract HIV/AIDS.
12 HIV/AIDS is preventable.
13 HIV/AIDS only affects men.
14 HIV/AIDS is more dangerous for certain racial or ethnic groups of people.
15 You will become infected if you are near or care for a person with HIV/AIDS.
16 Persons who have HIV always know it.
17 A person with HIV/AIDS would never knowingly infect someone else.

MULTIPLE CHOICE (check all that apply):

18 HIV/AIDS is spread by:
  a) unprotected vaginal, anal, or oral sex
  b) breathing the same air
  c) casual contact, like shaking hands
  d) using unsterilized needles
  e) playing contact sports with an infected person
  f) using the same eating or drinking implements as an infected person.

19 HIV/AIDS is best avoided by:
  a) abstinence from sexual activity
  b) abstinence from intravenous drug use
  c) using a latex condom and nonoxynl-9 the first time you have intercourse with a person

20 When you become intimate with a sexual partner, you may become infected with an STD from:
  a) your partner
  b) your partner's previous sexual partner
  c) the partners of your partner's previous sexual partner (confusing, isn't it?)

B. What Does the Bible Say About AIDS?

The short answer is nothing. AIDS was not known in the ancient world; but other dread diseases, like leprosy, were known, and we can make some comparisons. Have on hand a commentary to help your investigation.

✎ Form an even number of groups. Half should look up **Leviticus 13** and the other half **Leviticus 14**. Chapter 13 deals with the diagnosis and chapter 14 concerns the cleansing of various skin diseases, which are discussed collectively as leprosy.

✤ These chapters have tons of rules. Who oversees the regulations?
✤ Who is the modern equivalent to that person?
✤ What happens to a person who is deemed to be truly sick?
✤ What happens to a person who is deemed to be either not really sick or who is recovered?
✤ What reason is there for those rules? How do you feel about that?
✤ What modern situations come to mind as you study these passages?

➤ Persons infected with HIV/AIDS have been compared to the ancient lepers, who were considered unclean and who had to live outside the community. One reason for expelling lepers was that no one knew for sure how the disease was spread, and they were taking no chances.

✤ Knowing what we know about the means of infection for HIV, do you think this is a reasonable analogy?
✤ Should persons with HIV/AIDS be sent away from the religious community in particular or society in general? Why or why not?

➤ One thing is clear from these two chapters. This serious illness was very much the business of the religious community; and it affected the entire community, not just the priest who made the decisions.

✤ What is your church doing about AIDS?
✤ About persons with HIV/AIDS?

C. Discussion Starters

Review answers to the inventory

✎ After checking responses to the inventory, spend time clearing up myths and discussing the facts of HIV/AIDS. More information is found in the section "Just the Facts," pages 86-93.

Discuss the risk of certain behaviors

✎ Ask teens how many of them think their current behavior puts them at-risk and why they respond as they do. You may want to separate the males and females and have same-sex counselors deal with issues of behavior in the privacy of segregated groups. (See also the article on denial on page 24.)

Explore teens' responses and watch for mythical thinking or expressions, such as a self-concept of being stronger than a disease out there or statements like, "My partner loves me and wouldn't do anything to harm me."

Explore the implications of the long incubation period of HIV/AIDS

A person can be infected for several years, have no symptoms, not know of the infection, and thus put many people at risk.

✎ Ask teens to draw stick figures on a chart that shows how the chain of infection can spread. Use different colors or letters and other symbols to indicate the various pairings and behaviors of partners or participants, so that they have a graphic view of how pervasive HIV/AIDS is and continues to be. The chart should include the use of intravenous drugs too. For example, using eight participants:

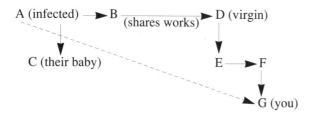

Stage 1: (A) is infected and has a sexual partner (B)
Stage 2: (A) and (B) have a baby (C)
Stage 3: (D) shares (B's) contaminated drug works
Stage 4: (D) (a virgin) and his/her first partner (E)
Stage 5: (E) has sexual partner (F)
Stage 6: Your boy/girlfriend (F) and you (G) as potential sexual partners

✎ Ask teens to imagine and discuss what happens when the persons in this graph have multiple partners. Some persons may think that if (F) is (G's) only partner that (G) must be safe. In reality, (G) is infected because of (A) and intervening partners.

Discuss with teens:

✤ After looking at this chart, what do you think "at-risk" means now?

✤ (E) told (F) truthfully that his/her only other partner (D) was a virgin. What assumptions would or could (E), (F), and (G) make from that statement? Can you rely on assumptions of safety? Why or why not?

Answers to the Inventory

1 False; HIV/AIDS is no respecter of age, sex, sexual orientation, race, or culture.
2 False; HIV/AIDS is contagious, but only under specific behavioral conditions, not by airborne germs.
3 True
4 False
5 False; a married, monogamous couple who are not infected will not contract HIV/AIDS from each other by sexual contact, but could through the use of contaminated needles.
6 False; see number 1.
7 False
8 True
9 False
10 False; not as of April 1993
11 True
12 True
13 and 14 False; HIV/AIDS is dangerous for EVERYONE.
15 False; the virus may take several weeks to several months to show up in testing, and a person can be without symptoms for as much as seven to ten years from the time of infection.
16 False
17 False; you must never assume that you are not at risk unless you absolutely and always refrain from at-risk behavior regarding sexual activity and intravenous drug use.
18 a and d
19 a and b. Until you know for a fact that you and your partner are not infected and do nothing to become infected, you must use adequate protection each and every time.
20 a, b, and c if anyone along the way is infected

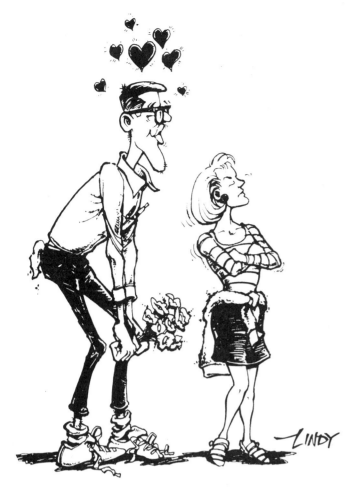

you're a virgin or not), here are a few tips that can make your choice easier:

➤ Surround yourself with friends who feel the way you do about not having sex right away.
➤ Think twice about dating or hanging out with people older than you.
➤ Double-date or go out in groups.
➤ Don't get in a car alone with anyone you don't trust.
➤ Don't go to a date's house when you'll be the only ones there.
➤ Don't take flirting too far.
➤ Don't drink alcohol or do drugs. Their effect may cause you to do things you normally wouldn't do—like have sex.
➤ Learn how to say no when it's necessary.

One teenager said she refused to have sex with the biggest hunk she ever went out with. Although she was extremely attracted to him, she felt that he only wanted to use her for sex, not a real relationship. "Having sex with him would have made me feel cheap," she says, "I think sex is the bonus to a loving relationship. So I said no. The funny thing is, it's two years since that happened and we're still in touch, still friends."   —*Eileen Nechas*

Reprinted from "HIV/AIDS and Other STD's," one of four theme issues from the series *Straight Talk: A Magazine for Teens TM* published by The Learning Partnership, Pleasantville, NY.

Saying No to Sex

"Everybody's having sex. I'm the only virgin left in my school."

This could be the biggest myth among teenagers today. And the pressure of wanting to "be like everybody else" is one of the main reasons many teens say "yes" when they really want to say "no" to sex.

It's normal to think about having sex and wonder what it would be like, says Jane Quinn, director of program services for Girls Clubs of America. But having sex too young, before you're emotionally ready, can be a disappointing experience. Some teenagers think sex will always be this way and therefore have a harder time developing good sexual relationships when they are more mature.

"Teenagers need to consider some important issues before they make the decision to have sex," says Quinn. Besides the risk of pregnancy, there's the chance of getting sexually transmitted diseases like HIV infection.

Teens who have sex at an early age also risk losing respect for themselves and their bodies. Will you disappoint your family, friends, and, most of all, yourself? Will you compromise your values? Will you feel guilty?

If you would like to abstain from sex for now (whether

For Further Reflection

Just saying no is not always easy, nor is it enough in some cases. Here are a series of helpful steps that can be added to make a no mean business. Can you think of others that have worked for you or someone else you know? These refer specifically to pressure to have sex, but they can be used elsewhere.

✎ Review these steps, then break into pairs to practice them. Just say no and . . .
➤ add an alternative activity: "I don't want to get so serious. We can have lots of fun with the whole crowd."
➤ add a reason: "I'm not going to have sex with you. The risk of infection with HIV/AIDS is too much to ask."
➤ confront the pressure: "I won't get that physical with you, and I don't appreciate your false accusation that I don't care for you."
➤ add movement: "I don't think we should go that far, and I won't stay here with you if you insist." Then leave, in a cab, if you have to.

Krista's Story

In the fall of 1990, Krista Blake was 18 and looking forward to her first year at Youngstown State University in Ohio. She and her boyfriend were talking about getting married. Her life, she says, was "basic, white-bread America." Then she went to the doctor, complaining about a backache, and found out she had the AIDS virus.

Blake had been infected with HIV, the virus that causes AIDS, two years earlier by an older boy, a hemophiliac. "He knew that he was infected, and he didn't tell me," she says. "And he didn't do anything to keep me from getting infected, either." When she first heard the diagnosis, Blake felt as though she had just walked into a brick wall. Suddenly, she couldn't envision her future. She found herself thinking things like "There are 50 states out there. I don't want to just live and die in Ohio." Her doctor sent her to University Hospital in Cleveland, 90 minutes from home, for treatment. She has taken AZT and is now on the new antiviral DDI. Although she needed frequent transfusions to counteract the effects of AZT, she is relatively healthy. "I am living with AIDS, not dying from AIDS," she says. "I do all of the same things I used to do. That doesn't mean I can run the Boston Marathon, but my mind is still 20." She reads everything from Danielle Steel to "Life 101," a popular advice book. She makes a point of going out at least once every day, even if it's just down to the park to watch a softball game. "It gets those juices moving," she says.

Still, she doesn't know how long her good health will last—a month, a year, five years. She doesn't make long-term commitments. Blake and her fiancé broke off their engagement, because, she says, "I love him enough that I want him to have his options for a life open." However, they are still very good friends. Blake also dropped out of school. "A bachelor's degree wouldn't do much for me," she says with a rueful laugh.

Since the spring of 1991, Blake has spent as many as four or five days a week doing the one thing she believes is really important—talking to other teens about HIV and how to avoid infection. The first thing the kids ask about is her sex life. "I don't have a sex life," she tells them, "but that's because I don't have any energy to have a sex life." The kids usually start laughing. Then she says: "I have just so much energy and I have to decide, do I come out here and talk to you, or do I have sex? I pick what's important, and you won." After one presentation, a student came up to Blake and told her: "I had an uncle who came home at Easter one year, and he had AIDS. This was in 1988. My mom was afraid. We didn't go see him. She wouldn't let us go. He died the next year, at Easter. I never got to say goodbye to my uncle. Would it be OK if I came up and gave you a hug?"

—Lucille Beachy

Why Did You Do This to Me?

Blake was infected by a young man who did not tell her he was HIV positive. Why would someone knowingly put another person at risk? Explore with teens the possible reasons and how they think they would feel in Krista's place.

Fear of rejection: Even though some infected persons are aware of the dangerous consequences of their behavior, they may be so fearful of rejection they won't reveal anything that could compromise their acceptance. "If you know I'm sick, you won't love me anymore."

Ignorance: Blake's partner was not ignorant of having the disease, but he could have been ignorant of how it is transmitted.

Apathy: Some infected persons may feel so low about their own situation that they feel there is nothing they can or need to do to help others.

Fatalism: Some infected persons, especially those in the statistically highest risk groups, may assume that all their potential partners are ill anyway and take no precautions to protect themselves or others.

Denial: The discovery of being infected is so devastating that one immediate response is denial. "This didn't/couldn't happen to me." The resulting behavior is acting as if the infection is not real or serious.

Lack of commitment: Some persons may assume that because their intended contact with another person lacks depth or commitment, they do not have to worry about the consequences of what they do. But "One time won't matter" does.

Anger: Rather than ignoring the facts, some infected persons may act out of anger or an attitude that says, "If I'm going to die, someone else is too."

Revenge: Some infected persons have deliberately infected as many others as they can to "punish" the world or a particular group of persons for their own illness.

For Further Reflection
Explore Some Key Points in Krista's Story

Not Being Able to Envision a Future

Have the teens make a list of all the things they expect to do in the next five, ten, and fifteen years. Ask them to rate each item according to its importance to them now, with 1 as very important and 5 as least important. Then give these directions.

✎ You are ill. These are your circumstances: frequent nausea and fevers, loss of appetite, low energy, poor concentration, occasional short-term hospitalization.

✎ Revise your list according to what you think you can accomplish. Make changes and adjustments based on your current circumstances. (Challenge unrealistic thinking.)

✎ Three years have passed and you are severely ill. (Describe some of the symptoms mentioned on page 86 for HIV infection. Point out that Krista reacted badly to her medication also.)

✎ Revise your list again.

Now lead a discussion of what attitudes, opinions, assumptions, or insights teens have gained or changed about the risk of HIV infection. Ask them also to talk about the effect their changed lives could have on their family and friends.

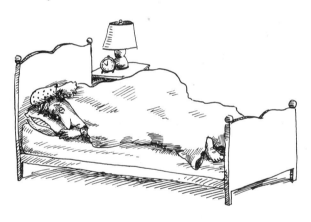

The Importance of Looking Ahead

Krista tries to look ahead instead of dwelling on what she can't change. Without denying her condition, she wants her life to count for something. A new priority is speaking to teens at school.

✎ Ask the teens to write on index cards the things they would want to ask her if she came to their school or church group. Address the concerns now that you can. Use the other cards as a basis for later discussion time after you have researched some more.

✤ Then ask: How can you offer support to someone like Krista? What impact does Krista's story have on you? Can you imagine yourself in her place?

A Constricted Social Life

Krista's story mentions several things about her social life—the decision to quit college, reading, going out each day, a broken engagement, her sex life, and her high school visits. One larger point in the story is that Krista doesn't have the energy to do everything she wants. To point out her situation, play the following game.

✎ Pass out small squares of paper to each person, two for every letter of their full name. These are "energy bits."

✎ Brainstorm and record a daily schedule of 12 or so everyday activities of most teens, assigning an "energy score" to each activity. For example, watching TV needs 1 energy bit, driving needs 4, a full school day needs 8, and so on.

✎ Gather everyone in a circle and place a basket for the energy bits in the center.

✎ Begin the daily schedule with the person with the most bits. Each person, in turn, will spend energy bits for each activity during the day, based on that person's total bits available, mandatory activities, and optional activities.

✎ When everyone's energy is spent, ask:

✤ How soon was your energy gone?

✤ What did you have to give up?

✤ How did it feel to see others keep going when you had to quit?

✤ How did it feel to watch others have to stop?

✤ If HIV infection can rob you of your life, what can you do to be sure you aren't infected? Will you follow through to protect yourself?

What Does the Bible Tell Us?

Have a commentary on hand to help understand the following passages of Scripture. Ask older teens to look up the Job passages and younger teens to look up the Scripture in Matthew. Everyone will answer the two questions.

Job was tested by a series of calamaties against him and his family. He had a hard time dealing with them, but eventually reaffirmed God's control and goodness.

✱ **Job 3:11-26—** Job's complaint about his misery.

✱ **Job 40:1-9—** The challenge by God to Job for his doubt and complaint.

✱ **Job 42:1-10—** Job's repentence and restoration.

Jesus announced to all that even though they (and we) had difficult circumstances to bear, he was and is with all persons to help them and to make the burden light.

✱ **Matthew 11:25-30—**Jesus will provide rest and help.

✤ What do these passages suggest about dealing with a devastating illness like AIDS?

✤ How do you think God and Jesus Christ lighten our painful burdens?

Tribute to a Friend
by Deva Hubbard

I had a dear friend named "Karl." "Karl" was one of the sweetest, most easy-going, happy people imaginable. I used to ask God why he had to take "Karl", but now I know that God did what God had to. I now think of it as a blessing to have had this experience, but it wasn't always like that.

"Karl" and his roommate were friends of my family for eleven years. "Karl" used to help my mom with her stereo equipment, and his roommate Carter used to help my mom with the computer. Our apartment doors were always open and we visited almost daily. I didn't really know what to think when I first found out that "Karl" had AIDS. I was eleven or twelve years old and AIDS wasn't that mainstream yet. I didn't know that much about it, but I did know that I wasn't in danger. I couldn't be in danger; we all loved each other too much. Nothing could happen, right?

Things were almost happy for a while. Everything went back to normal, and I forgot about it. Everyone was happy. Life was good. Suddenly "Karl" was fired from one of his jobs. His employer didn't say why, but we knew. His other employer seemed to be more understanding. "Karl's" colleagues also loved him, and they didn't let him go until he absolutely couldn't work anymore—about the time he lost the use of his arm and leg.

That was when it really hit me that "Karl" wasn't going to be around after a while. My mom always told me that I could make him happy, so whenever I could I would go over there to his apartment, which was across the hall from ours, to see him, usually to bring food, but sometimes just to bring a smile and a picture I had drawn.

The last two or so months of his life, I didn't see him. "Karl" was in the hospital most of the time. It wasn't that I didn't want to see him, because I did. I continued sending him pictures and flowers. It was more like I didn't want to see him the way he was—hooked up to machines, and all. I prayed to God every day that I'd wake up in the morning and there would be a cure and he would come home and everything would be all right, but some miracles take God time to accomplish.

"Karl" was a miracle in himself. He was always in good spirits; he never complained; he never bad-mouthed anyone; and he had a strong faith in God. That faith, I think, along with God's steadfast love is what kept him together so long. "Karl" was never angry or sad. He asked God for guidance, and it was given to him. If there is such a thing as an angel on earth, I believe "Karl" was one.

Even when "Karl" died, the Spirit was within him. It was within us also. Although we shed tears, everyone at his memorial service came away with a smile and a warm, happy feeling that "Karl" was where he was happiest—with his God. We were confident that his spirit would be looking down on us for the rest of our earthly days, and when our days were up, we'd see his ever-smiling face again and spend the rest of eternity with him.

This experience was very good for me. I was thirteen when "Karl" died, so I learned right away that AIDS and friends with AIDS were nothing to be scared of. I knew that cooking for them or with them wouldn't hurt me and that there was nothing better for an AIDS patient than a hug and a smile.

"Faith in God and faith in yourself are all you really need to get you through." That was the big lesson I learned from "Karl" and that I'm still learning from my friends who are HIV positive or who have AIDS. The Lord will pull you through and lead you to an eternity of peace and happiness.

This experience has also strengthened me considerably. It has helped me to care more, to understand more, and to love more. I can now be around people burdened with this horrible disease and know that God has a plan for each and every one of them. God's plan for me right now is to help these people in any way I can. For me, praying is the easiest thing. I know that my prayers are heard and that they will be answered, so I try not to worry.

I am confident that the Lord will deliver. Our Lord is an awesome Lord. All praise to God.

Deva Hubbard is fifteen years old and has lived in the Arts District of New York City all her life. Since receiving a call from God to do God's service almost three years ago, she has been willing to help as many people as are willing to accept God into their hearts.

For Further Reflection

Look at the Key Points in Deva's Tribute

We Weren't in Danger; We Loved Each Other

Deva learned that HIV/AIDS can dramatically change a relationship.

- Why did Deva think nothing could happen? Do you agree or disagree? Why?
- "Karl" was evidently a gay man. What else do you know about him? What does Deva think of him?
- Do you think there is a typical HIV/AIDS patient? (There isn't.) Why or why not?
- Deva's love of "Karl" is a healthy, affectionate love for a friend, not romantic love. What is the difference? What kind of love could put a person in danger of infection?

Learning About HIV/AIDS Early

- Deva was told about an adult friend's infection when she was a preteen. She is now 15. What are the advantages and disadvantages of talking to children and youth about HIV/AIDS?
- What do you think are the most effective ways of teaching children and teens about HIV/AIDS? teaching adults? What are the reasons for your answer?
- You are learning about HIV/AIDS now. What difference do you think this will make in your life? in your decisions?

HIV/AIDS Ruins Your Career

- "Karl" was fired from one job and had to leave the other one because of ill health. Do you think being fired because of sexual orientation or because of HIV/AIDS infection is fair? Why or why not?
- Can you become infected through casual contact with a coworker? What is the reason for your answer?
- Would you be willing to work with someone whom you know is HIV positive? Why or why not?
- If you were the person infected, would you think or feel differently about any of your responses?
- If a person is infected as a teenager, he or she may be too ill in early adulthood to think about, plan for, or pursue a career. What do you "want to be when you grow up"? Would you have time to prepare for and enjoy that career if you were infected?

Caring for Persons with HIV/AIDS

- What are the ways Deva helped care for and about "Karl"?
- Did her caring for "Karl" have any effect on Deva? What? Why?
- Think about someone you know who has HIV/AIDS or engages in behavior that puts him or her at risk for infection. What can you do or say to be a caring friend?

The Work of God Through the Holy Spirit

Deva makes several comments about how her faith in God affected her attitudes and behavior.

- What are some of the ways Deva says God was at work?
- Do you think God works that way? Why or why not?

Deva also talks about God's plan both during and after "Karl's" illness. For "Karl" (and apparently according to "Karl") the plan was healing in death; for her the plan is for ministry to others facing a future with HIV/AIDS. Look up the following Scriptures in the Bible and in a commentary to see what they say about such a plan.

- **Philippians 4:4-14**
- **Romans 8:1-2, 28, 31-35, 37-39**
- **John 14**
- **Mark 8:34—9:1**
- **Matthew 25:31-46**
- **Isaiah 58:5-11**

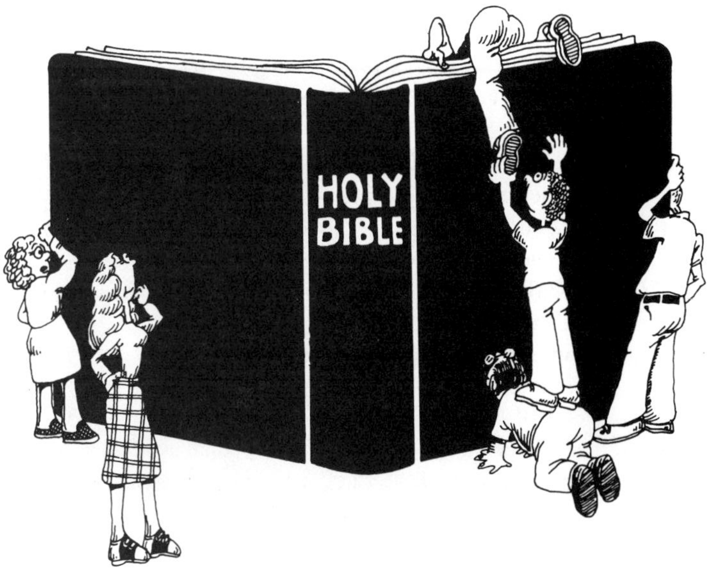

Hope's Story

Much of Hope's story is a string of painful memories:

She remembers being tucked into her bed as a 5-year-old and feeling snug under sheets and a comforter covered with cartoon pictures of Noah's ark. But in the past few years, the word "ark" has taken on an entirely new meaning for Hope, as her mother developed AIDS-related complex—known as ARC. The disease eventually progressed into AIDS, and Hope's mother died last September at age 49.

Hope, who is now 20, remembers the sadness of her father's death when she was 9 and the pronouncement she made to her mother soon afterward. "If you ever die," she told her, "I'll kill myself." Now her mother is gone, and that 11-year-old promise burns in her memory.

Hope remembers a day five years ago, when she opened a letter from the Santa Monica Hospital and became the first to learn that her mother had tested positive for HIV, the virus that causes AIDS. When her mother came into the room, Hope blurted, "I love you—I'm sorry," and threw her arms around her.

Hope remembers being on the phone a few months later and answering a call-waiting beep. "Is your mom there?" the new caller asked. "Yes, but I'm on the other line," Hope said. "Oh, that's okay. Just tell her Jay Morgan died." The caller had far too casually identified the man, an injection drug user, from whom Hope's mother had contracted HIV.

Hope remembers taking part in Los Angeles' annual Candlelight Vigil for AIDS two years ago, a giant group walk that started at the UCLA campus. As she and her mother hurried with a number of other people from their cars to the start of the march, two men passing by asked the group where they were going. Told about the vigil, the men sneered, "Oh, are you gay? Do you have AIDS? Are you going to die?"

"You never get used to it, but you deal with it," Hope says of her experiences. "You just do. I'm a survivor. I used to laugh at bad things a couple of years later. Now it's a couple of days later."

It's no wonder, though, that she's continually frustrated with her peers' ignorance about AIDS. "I don't care about losing friends anymore, because they don't care," she says with a sigh. "No one even thinks about the dangers of drugs or unprotected sex. They think they're invincible."

A few months before her mother died, Hope offered a vivid and sobering description of life with a person with AIDS. "It's being afraid to leave and being afraid to come home," she says. "It scares me, because I see this person who looks so different from what she used to look like. Sometimes she's ashamed of how she looks, so I tell her, 'Mom, you're beautiful. Look at me and see yourself.' It's hard. It's like, who's the parent? Sometimes I feel like she's my child and I'm this little mommy.

"I've learned about strength," Hope continues. "She's an example to me. Her disease forced me to stop thinking, 'You did this to yourself. It's not my problem, so I don't want to deal with it.' It forced me to be more compassionate. Sometimes I have to be stronger than I want to be."

But finally, when doctors summoned Hope to her mother's hospital bedside for the last time, there was no longer any need for her to be strong. The last few minutes of her mother's life are another memory that will stay with Hope forever. She laid down beside her, put her arms around her and rested her head on her mother's chest. "I knew I'd never have a chance to feel that again," Hope says.

—Jim Harmon

Reprinted from "HIV/AIDS and Other STD's," one of four theme issues from the series *Straight Talk: A Magazine for Teens TM* published by The Learning Partnership, Pleasantville, NY.

PHOTO BY JIM WHITMER

For Further Reflection on Hope's Story

Explore some of the key points in Hope's story by using these discussion starters.

Dealing with Cruel and Cavalier Feelings and Actions of Others

Hope reports two incidents in which someone was either casual or cruel regarding her feelings—the phone caller and the passersby at the vigil.

✎ Brainstorm some ways a person can respond and cope with those kinds of actions. Decide which suggestions are mature and healthy ones and why.

✎ Assign clusters of two or three persons in which one takes the role of a teen in Hope's situation, another is the antagonist creating the situation, and a third person (if needed) is one to whom the teen can turn.

Have each small group act out a healthy response to a similar situation.

✎ As a whole group, review what was portrayed and ways teens can both care for themselves or others who are put down somehow because of HIV/AIDS.

The Parent-Child Relationship

Hope's story has an interesting twist in that we are less likely to expect parents to have to confess the results of at-risk behavior to their children than the other way around.

- Hope found out first about her mother's infection. She reports two different reactions. What are they?
- How do you expect your parents to conduct their personal lives? Why?
- What kind of model or example do you want your parents to be? Why?
- What support and encouragement can you provide for them?

Hope also discovered that as her mother became more ill there were times when their roles reversed and she became a "little mommy" to her mother.

- In what ways did Hope become like a mother to her mother?
- What did Hope learn?

Losing Both Parents

Many teens have dealt with the pain of separation from a parent due to divorce, but fewer will have lost a parent who died. Even fewer can relate to the death of both parents.

- To help teens try to grasp this, look for what Hope says regarding these losses. What memories does she have? What fears? What disappointments?
- What signs might you notice in a person who is struggling with a fatal illness in the family? What issues are added when that illness is HIV-related?
- What can teens do to offer support or to seek support?

Knowing the Truth, Speaking the Truth

Hope expresses frustration and resignation that other teens and young adults are so ignorant or unconcerned about the causes and dangers of HIV/AIDS. She has painful, firsthand knowledge of the devastation; she knows the awful truth about AIDS. She yearns for others to listen.

Check out these Scriptures in your Bible and in a Bible commentary to see what the Bible says about telling the truth, especially truth others don't seem to want to hear.

❇ **Jeremiah 37:17—38:6, 14-16**; Should Jeremiah give up?

❇ **Mark 6:6b-13**; Sometimes you have to leave where you are not wanted. How hard should you keep trying and what are the consequences if you give up?

❇ **John 8:25-38**; How can the truth make you free? How will faith in God help a person with HIV/AIDS?

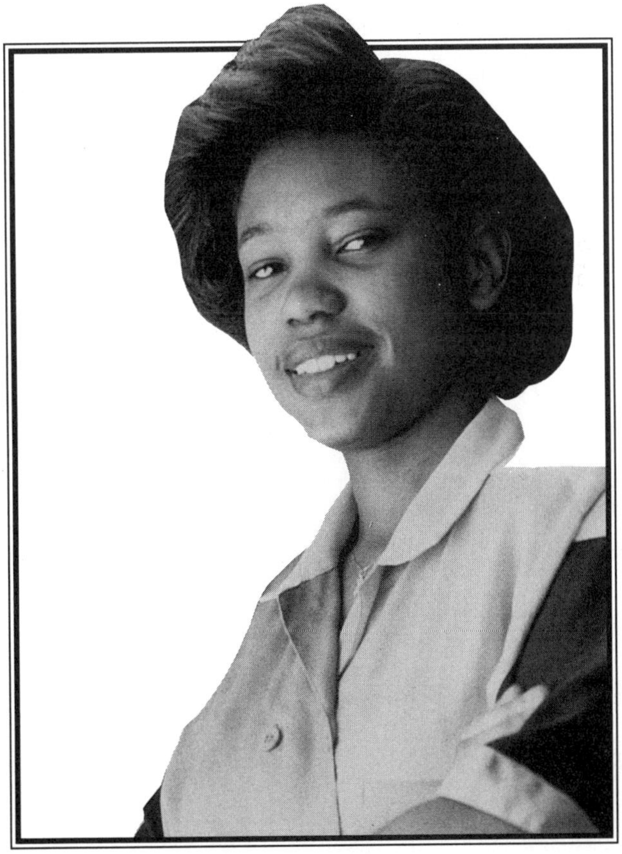

PHOTO BY JIM WHITMER

AIDS and Drugs:
What You Should Know

Michelle, a 19-year-old college sophomore, has it all: brains, good looks, a great personality, a loving family—and AIDS. She got the deadly virus from her boyfriend, Rick.

One time when Rick got high at a party, a friend talked him into shooting cocaine. His friend shot up first, then passed the needle and syringe to Rick.

Rick didn't know his friend was infected with HIV. A tiny bit of contaminated blood remained in the needle and got into Rick's bloodstream. That's all it took to pass the virus to Rick, and then to Michelle because they had sex without a condom.

Rick and Michelle's story depicts the sad reality of how drug use can lead to AIDS. The facts are simple: Sharing a drug needle or syringe with a person who has HIV places you at risk of being infected. So does having sex with a person who uses injection drugs like heroin, speed or steroids. In fact, you can catch other STDs, such as hepatitis B, through these behaviors, too.

The Risk of Sharing Needles

One way HIV, the virus that causes AIDS, is spread is when it enters a person's bloodstream. When an infected person shoots drugs, blood can be trapped in the needle, then injected into the bloodstream of the next person who uses the needle. Even the smallest amount of blood left in a used needle or syringe can contain HIV. Sharing needles puts you and anyone you have sex with at risk for infection.

Reducing your exposure to HIV is one good reason to avoid doing drugs. Here are accurate answers to a few common myths about drug use, HIV and AIDS:

MYTH: "If I don't shoot drugs or share needles, I can't get AIDS from taking drugs, right?"

FACT: Sharing drug needles or syringes with a person who's infected with HIV exposes you to the virus. But other kinds of drugs, including alcohol, can also cause problems. Under the influence of drugs, it's harder to think clearly. Your judgment becomes clouded, and you can fool yourself into feeling you're more in control than you really are. You could be exposed to HIV while doing things you wouldn't otherwise do—-like sharing needles or having unprotected sex.

MYTH: "I can tell by looking if someone shoots drugs or has AIDS. If I don't have sex with those people, I'll be safe."

FACT: You can't assume that someone hasn't experi-

mented with injection drugs or isn't infected with HIV just because he or she doesn't fit the stereotype of a "typical" drug user. A person can be infected with HIV without showing any symptoms—and possibly without even knowing that he or she is infected.

The bottom line: If you have sex, always practice safer sex. And never share needles. Don't rely on other people's assurances about their health—always protect yourself.

MYTH: "It can't happen to me. Only gay guys and drug addicts get AIDS."

FACT: It's not who you are but what you do that determines whether you'll get infected with HIV. The virus can affect anyone—of any age, race, ethnic background or sexual orientation—who engages in risky behavior, such as having unprotected sex (sex without a condom) or sharing a needle with an infected person.

Through June 1991, more than 37,000 Americans between the ages of 13 and 29 have been diagnosed with AIDS, and many of them became infected as teenagers.

——Elizabeth Mauro

The Other Needles

Because injection drug use is a well-known transmission route for HIV, the virus that causes AIDS, you may wonder: "What about other needles? What if I get my ears pierced? Or give blood? Can I get STDs from those needles?"

"Other needles" are any needles used to puncture skin. But needles do not automatically cause the spread of HIV. The transmission of STDs is only possible when a needle that is not sterilized properly is used by an infected person and then a non-infected person. So when do you have to worry about the other needles? To get answers to our questions, we went straight to an expert. Dr. Robert Johnson, the director of adolescent medicine at New Jersey School of Medicine, offered this information:

Giving blood (blood donation): Donating blood in the U.S. poses no STD risk because the needles are sterile and disposable and are thrown away immediately after they're used. "One of the points we've tried to make over and over is that there's no risk of getting AIDS from giving blood," Dr. Johnson says.

Tattooing: Risky business.
"This is dangerous because tattooers sometimes use the same needles on various people," Dr. Johnson says. Although he can recall only one case of AIDS that has

been linked to tattooing, Dr. Johnson believes tattooing involves a definite risk. If you must get a tattoo, make sure the needles are sterile.

Acupuncture: This is the ancient Chinese practice of relieving pain or disease with the use of needles. If the needles used are sterile, Dr. Johnson does not believe there is a risk for getting viral STDs, as long as the acupuncturist is reputable and the needles are maintained properly.

Vaccination: These shots are given to prevent diseases such as measles, tetanus and diphtheria, and they're important to maintaining good health. "Vaccinations do not transmit HIV," Dr. Johnson says. "Vaccinations are approached in the same way as blood donations—a new needle is used for every person—so you cannot get HIV."

Ear piercing: "There is virtually no risk involved in ear piercing when it's done in a regular clinic setting or at a mall and the needle is sterile," says Dr. Johnson. "But it becomes risky when teenagers do it themselves and share needles."

Blood transfusion: This is a medical procedure in which a person receives someone else's blood. It's usually performed in an emergency, often in a life-or-death situation. "Because all blood is tested for HIV before it is given to someone else, the possibility of someone getting HIV from a transfusion is extremely slim." Dr. Johnson says.

—Mary K. Cassidy

Steroids: Triple Trouble

To try to make themselves superhuman, many teenage athletes turn to steroids, synthetic drugs that mimic the male hormone testosterone. These drugs are said to enhance strength and muscle-building ability, but they're not without risks:

- ➤ In the short term, steroids provide the body with a jolt of aggressiveness that causes many users to experience erratic and sometimes psychotic or suicidal behavior.
- ➤ Prolonged use of steroids carries a long list of health risks—not the least among them being sterility, kidney failure, cancer and heart disease.
- ➤ Now add the latest threat: HIV infection.

Because steroids are illegal, they're an extremely profitable item on the black market. More than half the steroids used are injectable, making the market for needles equally big. And it's not uncommon for pushers to repackage used needles and resell them.

The resiliency of a strong body has helped many athletes achieve their dreams. Steroids, with their increased risk of HIV infection and AIDS, are a surefire way to turn those dreams into nightmares.

—Laura Dayton

Reprinted from "HIV/AIDS and Other STD's," one of four theme issues from the series *Straight Talk: A Magazine for Teens TM* published by The Learning Partnership, Pleasantville, NY.

For Further Reflection

Disease Transmission During Injection Drug Use

HIV can be passed during injection drug use and then to sexual partners of those drug users.

- ✤ How is HIV transmitted during drug use? What other diseases can you catch?
- ✤ How much do you know about those diseases?
- ✤ How many ways do you know to prevent the spread of disease during injection drug use? What do you think is the best way? Why?
- ✤ Is risking using a contaminated needle worth the danger of contracting an STD, especially a fatal one?

What About Other Needles?

You don't have to be a junkie to be infected by a contaminated needle.

- ✤ What are the other needles?
- ✤ How can you protect yourself?
- ✤ What would you say to a friend who is not taking any precautions?

Dealing With the Myths

Examine the three myths that reflect the "It can't happen to me" attitude.

- ✤ Have you accepted any of those myths as truth?
- ✤ After knowing the facts, can you still accept that kind of mythical thinking? Why or why not?
- ✤ What would you say to a friend who gives you one of those excuses?

After discussing possible responses to this third question, break up into pairs and practice having conversations that urge teens to be responsible.

What Can the Bible Tell Us?

Look up these passages in the Bible and in a commentary. What do they say about being responsible?

- ❇ **Deuteronomy 5:28-33**
- ❇ **Romans 12:1-2**
- ❇ **1 Corinthians 6:15-20**

Kaye and Wally's Stories

We Hear From Kaye

Aids also kills dreams.

At 18, Kaye Brown was ready for the world. The bubbly honor student was looking forward to life in the army. Last March, she signed up at a recruiting office in Houston and took a mandatory AIDS test. A week later she learned she was HIV-positive, and the world was no longer a sure thing. "I was really, really angry," she says. "My career had been snatched away from me."

Though doctors estimated that she had contracted the virus recently, they recommended that she get in touch with anyone she had had sex with in the previous year. The list was long. "It was easy for me to list the guys I had slept with," she says, "but when I counted 24, I was like, gosh!" Brown chose to tell them personally. One former partner said, "But you don't look like you're that way." Brown shot back, "What is *that way*? HIV doesn't mean that I'm dirty or low. It just means I made a mistake." Her boyfriend couldn't cope with the news, and they split up. Not one man was willing to be tested. "They were too scared," Brown says.

Brown blames only herself; she never insisted on condoms. "It makes me angry that I allowed this to happen," she says. "Choices I made have stolen away the choices that I might have had in the future." Now she's turning her anger to good use by working at the AIDS Foundation Houston Inc., talking to teens. "Kids see people who have HIV as bad," she says, "I'm out there to prove that it does happen to good, everyday people." Most teenagers, says Brown, won't practice safe sex unless someone really close to them becomes ill. HIV, she tells them, "doesn't discriminate. It doesn't care how old you are or who you are." She refuses to put her life on hold, and next fall she'll attend Texas Southern University. She gobbles up romance novels ("If you can't live it, read it," she jokes) and lives a day at a time: "That way, worry won't kill me before HIV does." AIDS, she says, has given her a purpose: "I feel responsible for educating other young people. That's my big mission; that's why I'm here."

And Now From Wally

Getting a driver's license was a liberating experience for 16-year-old Wally Hansen, who grew up in a household so "normal [it was] almost like 'Leave It to Beaver'." He and some buddies in suburban Pinole, Calif., would cut classes and drive to the woods near a gay beach in San Francisco, where they would "frolic" with each other and the men they met there. Hansen never considered using a condom—this was the mid-'80s, when safe sex meant not getting caught by your parents.

Hansen eventually joined the air force. But in 1987, he was discharged after the service discovered he was a homosexual. Routine exit exams revealed the presence of the AIDS virus. Hansen, now 24, is almost certain he was first exposed to HIV during his hooky-playing days. Had he known about the growing epidemic, he says, he might have altered his behavior. He is convinced that education is the key to stopping the spread of AIDS among young people. The effort, he says, should begin in junior high. And since teenagers "are going to have sex no matter what," it's important, "especially in high school, to hand out condoms, anything." Hansen, an administrative assistant at the Bay Area Reporter, a gay paper in San Francisco, is active in the AIDS war. For two years he was a driver for Rubbermen, an organization that donates condoms to city bars, and now volunteers at AIDS fund-raisers.

But when it comes to his own health—and sometimes that of others—Hansen is reckless. He says he has used speed intermittently for two years. Though he knows that unprotected sex brings the risk of more infections with more strains of the AIDS virus, he doesn't always use a condom. He admits that many of his peers who are HIV-positive don't always inform their partners of their condition, on the assumption that they are infected, too. Some may see it as the behavior of the doomed, but to Hansen, "it basically comes down to what you think it's worth." He insists he wouldn't be happy if he restricted his activities. "I can only think positively. I do anything I want. I feel like I'd do more damage to myself by stressing my system out of worry." His family has taken his illness in stride. "My mom and dad told me they may not love the things I do," says Hansen, "but they love me." And that, sad to say, makes him luckier than many.

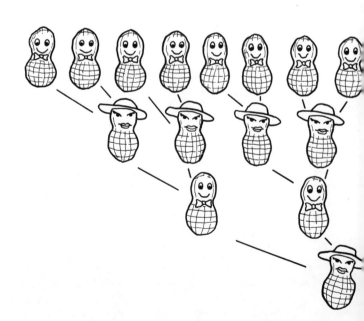

For Further Reflection on Kaye and Wally's Stories

Review the key points of Kaye and Wally's stories by using the following discussion starters for conversation or reflection.

Kaye's Story

Feelings at Discovery

Anger is a common reaction to terrible news, both at the time of discovery and later.

✤ Why was Kaye angry?

✤ What has she lost?

✤ How do you think you would feel in Kaye's circumstances? Why?

Multiple Sex Partners

Kaye accepted the responsibility to notify her sex partners and was surprised to realize she had had twenty-four in the previous year. She told all of them personally.

✤ Do you think having multiple sex partners increases a person's risk of infection? Why or why not?

✤ Why do you think someone would be willing to have so many different partners?

✎ Try this roleplay activity if you think your teens can handle it. Divide the teens into groups of four or five. Ask for a volunteer to roleplay a person who is HIV-positive. He or she will then tell each other person individually how he or she could have passed on the infection to that person. Each person who hears the news may react in whatever way comes to mind (within limits).

✤ How did it feel to have to confess? Name all your feelings.

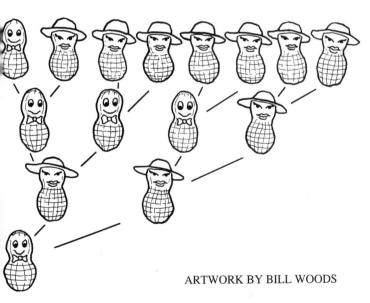

ARTWORK BY BILL WOODS

✤ How did it feel to be told you might be infected too? Name all your feelings.

✤ In your own mind, decide if your current behavior could actually put you in this position one day. If you are engaging in risky behavior, is it worth it? If you think so, why?

✤ Would you be willing to be tested? Why or why not?

Be sure to debrief the teens so that this exercise encourages teens to be safe and responsible, rather than to be reckless and secretive.

Wally's Story

Changing Definition of "Safe Sex"

There has been a shift in attitude over the years about sexual activity.

✤ What does Wally suggest is the "old" definition of safe sex? Do you agree? Why or why not?

✤ What is your current idea of safe sex?

✤ Do you think teens pay attention to that definition and follow through in practice? Why or why not?

Teen Education and Condom Distribution

Wally is convinced that HIV/AIDS education needs to begin with early teens. Education and information may have helped him make different decisions. But he also thinks that teenagers "are going to have sex no matter what."

✤ Do you agree with him? Why or why not?

✤ What difference is your own HIV/AIDS education making in your life?

✤ What do you think is the answer to the AIDS crisis? Is condom distribution the answer? Explain your responses.

"I Do Anything I Want"

In the last paragraph, Wally reveals something about his value system as shown in his reckless behavior.

✤ What is Wally doing and not doing that seems reckless to you?

✤ What do you think are Wally's values? Do you share any of his values? Why or why not?

✤ What do his values seem to say about caring for others? for himself?

✤ How do you feel about those values? Name your feelings.

What Does the Bible Say?

Look up these Scriptures in the Bible and in a commentary to see what they say about our interactions with others. Compare and contrast the biblical message with Kaye and Wally's stories.

✣ **John 15:1-17;** what does it mean to love one another?

✣ **Colossians 3:1-17;** can anyone be that "good"?

✣ **Exodus 20:13;** if someone infects you with HIV, is that person a murderer when you die?

I Have AIDS, and It's Terrible: An Interview with "John"

by Jeff Buck

Jeff: John, how old were you when you found out you were infected?

"John": I was 20 years old.

Jeff: How did you take the news?

"John": When the nurse told me the results, it was like someone had taken a stake and rammed it right through my chest.

Jeff: Did you ever consider that this disease might be a possibility?

"John": I honestly thought it would never happen. I always thought it was someone else's problem.

Jeff: How did your family and friends respond?

"John": Well, my family hasn't had a chance to respond yet because I have not told them. Well, let's just say it is a great fear in my life right now telling my family.

Jeff: Are you experiencing any sickness now?

"John": No, I feel very fortunate because I was diagnosed very early in the stages of the disease. I haven't had any of the symptoms.

Jeff: Would some people use that information to deny they have the disease completely?

"John": It is really hard. I sometimes feel like I really don't know what it is like because I can't feel it. The only thing that is overwhelming to me is that I wake up knowing that there is something there. There is like that black cloud. In the back of your mind it is there and affects you everyday.

Jeff: What would you say to teenagers right now to express to them to get their attention and say "Look, this is serious"?

"John": I would like to say that I was someone who dated regularly and was an average student. I had a lot of friends in high school. High school was a good time for me. But it happened to me, and it happened easily. And it can happen to anybody else. What I tell people is to *assume everyone is HIV positive.* If that doesn't put enough fear into your mind that if you are going to have sex, you'll use a condom, then hopefully it will put enough fear in your mind that you just won't have sex.

Everyone thinks they are getting a cure, but is there a cure out there? Well, no one has seen it yet. Everyone hears these rumors that they are going to come up with a cure or with something to stabilize it like they do with diabetes. Well, we haven't seen that yet, and it will still mean to take precautions. I honestly don't see a cure within my lifetime. I know people who have really considered ending their own life because of this.

For Further Reflection

Think about or discuss these questions:

✤ Do you think "John" was right in not telling his parents he is HIV positive? Why or why not?

✤ Do you think his parents would want to know? What about your parents?

✤ What do you think Jesus would say to "John"? to his parents?

✤ Describe "John's" hope for the future now. What hope could Jesus offer?

✤ "John" suggests that some people have considered suicide at some point following their diagnosis as HIV positive. What are your thoughts on that? Why do you hold those thoughts or opinions? Do you think you would feel differently if you contracted HIV? How do you think the community of faith could/should/would respond to a suicide attempt (or success) by a person with HIV/AIDS? Why do you think so?

✤ "John" mentions first using a condom and then abstinence as a means of protection. Would that be your order of priority? What does your faith suggest?

✤ Read the Parable of the Lost Son (**Luke 15:11-32**). Have the lost son come home with AIDS. Do you think the behavior of the father and the brother would change? Why or why not? What is the message for "John" in this parable? What is the message for us?

Rev. Jeff Buck has been involved with youth ministry in the local church, district, and conference level working particularly to help equip and motivate adults so that they can lead youth in faith and discipleship. Jeff presently serves as Associate Pastor at Castleton United Methodist Church in Indianapolis, Indiana. Jeff and his wife Julie have two daughters, Sarah and Anna.

Coping With Grief

by Yvonne Howze

As I write this article, a young friend of mine lies dying from complications resulting from HIV infection. I think about his bright mind, his excitement about the future, and his smile that always seems to light up a room. I think of his love for God, the church, and the people of God. As I begin to realize that the world will not experience the richness of his dreams, I feel sad. We will miss him. Family, church members, classmates, friends—we will all miss him. In fact, we have already begun missing him. We grieve not only for him, but also for the potential we will lose with his death.

Death is an experience of loss, but death is not the only loss that people feel. Everyday living is filled with experiences involving "little deaths." Anytime something or someone of value is taken from us, we experience loss. Grief is an important and normal reaction to the experience of loss. Any loss that we experience is upsetting to us, but death, particularly the death of someone we really care about, disrupts our lives and sets off the grieving process.

Stages of Grief

Grief is a process during which a person gives up that which is lost. There are several stages to the grieving process. Each stage must be gone through at the person's own pace if he or she is to be reestablished into the fullness of life in a positive manner. Here is a general outline of the stages of grief.

The first stage of grief is shock. When we learn of the death of a loved one, our grief begins. Everything screams NO to death. Shock is followed by denial. At this stage, words are of little comfort, and the grieving person may withdraw into himself or herself, or have outbreaks in behavior in an attempt to deal with the loss itself.

The second stage is characterized by disorganization and is seen as being out of touch with everyday activities, or as general confusion. In this stage the grieving person may be unable to make or carry out decisions.

The third stage is a deeply emotional one as the griever struggles between fantasy and the reality of the loss. During this time, a person may experience feelings of guilt, anger, and helplessness. In an attempt to ease the pain, the griever may also begin to view the person who died as a saint who could do no wrong.

The final stage is acceptance. The grieving person begins to accept the loss and starts the steps to giving up the emotional attachments to the one who has died. This does not mean that the grieving person will never think of the deceased person again, but she or he begins a hopeful look toward the future; hope without the physical presence of a loved one who has died.

Grief and AIDS

In the case of AIDS, grief begins when one finds out that she or he is HIV positive. Most young people have not given any thought to dying. It is just not "supposed to happen this way." After all, for most young people, death is what happens to the very sick or very old.

This is a difficult time also for parents. Parents commonly assume that their children will bury them and not the other way around. For parents, there is a sense of grief not only for the child, but also for the loss of connection with the future of their child. One of the double tragedies of AIDS for young people is that they have just begun to enter the adventure of an adult life when they must learn to come to grips with an early death. The psychological and developmental demands are heavy burdens for teens and their families.

Besides the possibility of an early death, the experience of grief for the person with AIDS comes from many sources. Many teenagers begin to identify goals and dreams for their future when they are 20, 30, or maybe 40 years old. The diagnosis of AIDS means the end of planning for a career later in one's adult life. It is hard to come to grips with AIDS in one's own life while realizing that through sexual contact or needle sharing, a friend or loved one may have also become infected. In this case, grief is mixed with fear and anxiety.

Because of the way a person gets the disease, AIDS sets in motion feelings of shame and guilt that cause many persons to try as hard as possible to keep this illness a secret. Persons with AIDS and their families will go to great lengths not to talk about this illness because they are trying to protect themselves from rejection by others. Feelings of shame and guilt often keep persons with AIDS and their families from turning to the church and others for support during the grieving process.

Caring for the Young Person with AIDS

Medical experts tell us that no one dies from AIDS itself but from *opportunistic illnesses* that result from a weakened immune system. When a doctor tells a person that she or he has AIDS, sooner or later he or she will die. In her work, Dr. Elisabeth Kübler-Ross identified five attitudes of dying persons. These attitudes are similar to but not the same as the stages of the grieving process. A person may not follow these attitudes (phases) in this given order; nevertheless, it is helpful for us to understand the phases dying persons go through. Kübler-Ross lists these attitudes as:

(1) **Denial**: A reaction that says "Not me!" and is common among those who learn that they have a disease that will result in their death.

(2) **Anger**: For the person with AIDS, anger is everywhere. Feelings of rage are often directed toward God. There is a general feeling of anger that others will remain healthy and the person with AIDS will die.

(3) Bargaining: The person accepts the facts about the illness and death but attempts to bargain, usually with God, for more time.

(4) Depression: With this attitude, one mourns things done, mistakes made, and wrongs committed. Here the dying person begins to prepare for death.

(5) Acceptance: This final attitude is marked by a sense of "It's all right" and seems to indicate that the person has made peace with others, self, and God.

Death is a mystery. Those suffering from AIDS experience the mystery of death in several ways. As a result of rejection, guilt, and shame, they experience the pain of their infection being made public and the death of their place in the family or community. Persons with AIDS also experience the sting of fear as they face the likelihood of their physical death. As we journey with persons living and dying with AIDS, we can create a space of safety for them as they explore their questions about life and death; and we can assure them that they are persons of worth and dignity as we surround them with the embrace of God's love.

For Further Reflection

Use the following exercises to reflect on the key points of the article.

Allow persons an opportunity to get a sense of the grief experienced by those facing loss.

Distribute pieces of paper and pencils to group members. Ask them to breathe deeply and regularly for a minute to help them settle in. Then ask them to list the following things on their paper:

- ✎ The most valuable (expensive) material possession they own (coat, jewelry—anything that they could sell).
- ✎ Other than God or themselves, the name of the most important person in their life.
- ✎ A hobby or other activity they truly enjoy.
- ✎ A secret about themselves that they have not told anybody.

Remind them that no one will see this paper so they can be completely honest. Then read the following story slowly to give time for listeners to consider the events and to do what the story asks. Suggest that they close their eyes when they are listening.

- ✎ You have been in an automobile accident. You have been rushed to the hospital. The doctors worked very hard and were able to save your life, but you can't wake up from the surgery. You are in a coma. Two days pass; two weeks pass; two months pass, and you are still in this coma. Finally, after six months in this coma, your most expensive possession has to be sold because there is a need for the money. (*Mark off list.*)

- ✎ You are still in this coma. After nine months, the strain becomes too much and the most important person in your life no longer comes to the hospital. (*Mark off list.*)

- ✎ Because you are in this coma, you can no longer enjoy your favorite hobby. (*Mark off list.*)

- ✎ The reason you were in the wreck is because your deep secret was discovered. You couldn't keep it a secret any longer. You were so upset that you weren't paying attention and ran out (or drove) in front of another car. You accidentally did this to yourself, and you may never get another chance to be more careful the next time.

- ✎ Now open your eyes and say in one word what you feel. (Lost, grief, hurt, sorrow, despair, panic, alone, anger, and frustrated may be some words you will hear.) Allow time for teens to talk about their feelings and how they think persons with HIV/AIDS might feel.

Discuss how teens can support others who are grieving.
- ✤ Look back at the stages of grief and the stages of dying. Discuss with teens when and how they think they can interact with someone who is grieving and when they should hold back. Consider the reasons.
- ✤ Sometimes grieving persons and their friends want to talk, but don't know how to get started. Each is waiting for the other to begin. What are some ways to recognize when you can start a conversation and what you might say?

How Can the Bible Help?

The Bible has numerous passages that affirm the goodness of God and God's presence in the time of trouble, including grieving. However, these affirmations of God's presence in the midst of suffering are difficult to learn in the midst of pain. We are much better prepared to cope with grief if we have previously cultivated the depth of faith that assures us of God's presence at all times and in all circumstances.

Look over one or more of the following passages, considering how they can bring comfort to someone who is grieving. Have a commentary on hand to help you understand the passages. The questions that follow do not necessarily connect to each Scripture passage.

❇ **Psalm 130**: We call to God from the depth of pain and God comforts and redeems us. We can hope in the Lord.

❇ **Lamentations 3:22-33**: God's steadfast love is abundant, and God does not willingly cause us grief.

❇ **John 16:16-24**: Jesus will die soon and his disciples will grieve, but their grief will be turned to joy because Jesus will see them again.

Use these questions to reflect on or to discuss the passages.

- What are ways you think God can redeem illness? (for example, a person with HIV turns his or her attention to educating others)
- What are ways that God can redeem death?
- What are your images of death? Are any of those images positive? (such as relief from suffering)
- What does the passage say about God and God's relationship to God's people?
- What do you think it means to "wait for the Lord"?
- What are the key words or phrases that offer hope?
- Jesus understood human grieving because he had the experience. He was not immune to any of the emotions faced by all persons. Why do you think he said that grief would turn to joy?
- What are some things we can ask God in the midst of grief that, when God gives it, will bring joy?

Yvonne Billingsley Howze is the Assistant Pastor of Payne Chapel AME Church, Nashville, TN. She also serves as Director for Project TEACH, an HIV/AIDS Education Awareness and Support ministry of Payne Chapel. The Reverend Howze is a native of Birmingham, AL, is married to Roy Howze, and is the mother of three children. She is currently completing her studies for the Doctor of Ministry degree at Vanderbilt University.

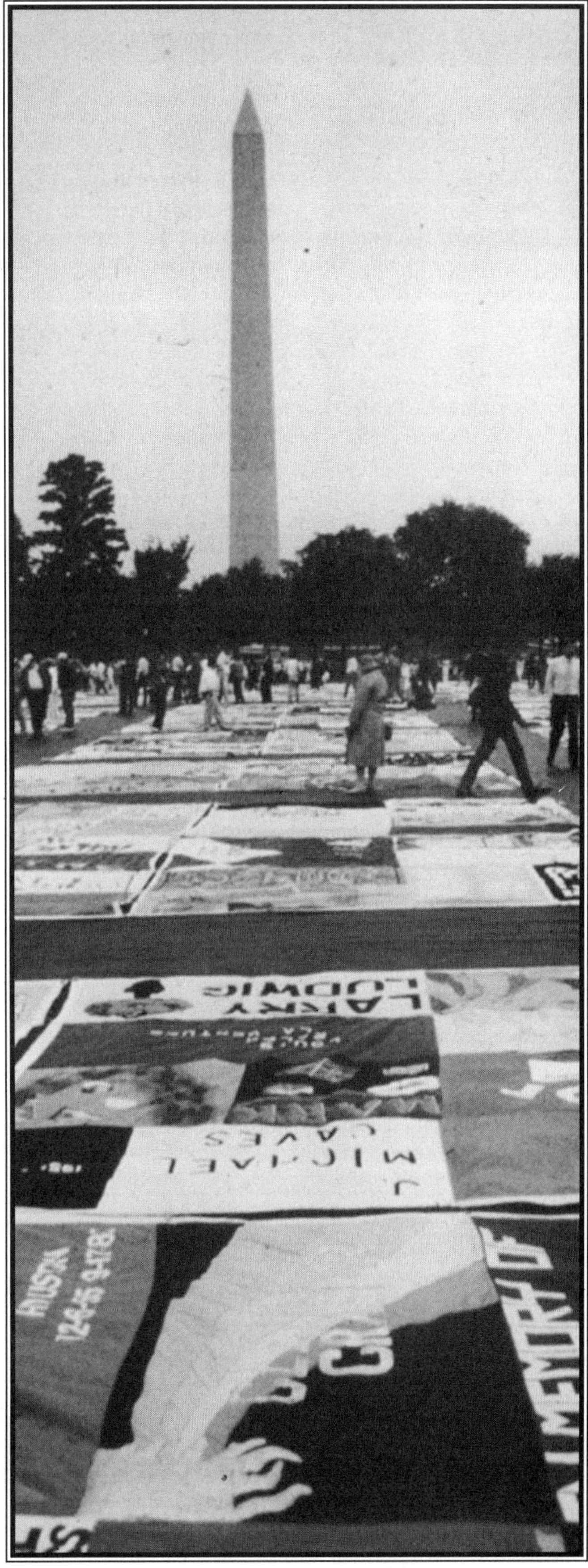

PHOTO BY CATHIE LYONS

Denial By Teens: See No Evil; Hear No Evil; Speak No Evil

by Jeff Buck

The Problem

A speaker who is HIV positive was invited to meet with a group of senior high students as part of their school's AIDS Awareness training. During the meeting, the speaker noticed a young woman who was obviously bored. So he finally asked her, "Aren't you afraid of getting HIV?"

"I'll never get it," she said.

The speaker said, "Good, but tell the class why."

She replied, "I am monogamous."

"OK, but tell the class what monogamy means."

"I just have sex with one person at a time. I don't do group sex!"

"How did you get that definition of monogamy?"

"Well, my sister had mononucleosis, and I was told that *mono* means *one*. So if I don't do group sex, but just have sex with one person at a time, I can't get AIDS."

In other words, this young woman did what many people do. She determined her own definition and then based her behavior on her incorrect assumption. This kind of reasoning leads to the attitude that says, "It can't happen to me!"

In a school system with an excellent program for HIV/AIDS education, one teenager said, "I can't get it because I am on the pill." She incorrectly assumes that her precautions to prevent pregnancy are enough to protect her from HIV. They aren't.

The Bases for Denial

Since 1981 when the Centers for Disease Control held a press conference announcing the discovery of AIDS, we have heard the myths and stigma of AIDS. I am sure you have heard that AIDS is a "gay" virus, that it is an injection drug user's virus. It is "their" problem. It is too easy to believe that "if I am not one of 'them,' I won't get AIDS."

An 18-year-old young man was at a party one night. All the guys decided to pierce their ears. They used one needle. Someone in that group was HIV positive, and his blood on that needle infected this young man as it was passed.

AIDS is a catchable, infectious disease from *anybody* who is HIV positive. The virus within one person's bodily fluids is transmitted to another by birth, by blood, or by the mingling of bodily fluids in the sexual act.

A doctor talking with a group of senior high's said, "You should not have intimate sexual activity with anyone whose past sexual history you do not know. Also, you should not have sex unless you know the sexual history of all their partners."

One of the guys was thinking this over and he said "Doc, it's a Saturday night, and I got the family car, and I am going out with a new woman. We drive to a dark place. I put my arm around her. And are you saying to me the first thing I should whisper into her ear is: 'tell me about all of your sexual activity and the activity of your past partners?'"

And the doctor said, "You should be worried that she hasn't already asked you!"

Sometimes other values and taboos are the root of the problem. When men value a "macho" attitude toward life in general and women in particular, not only are they prone to deny that they could be infected, but they do not use any protection either.

When a family system is constructed on values of family and personal honor, it does not tolerate well the idea that a family member could abandon the strong family ethics and engage in at-risk behavior. "It can't happen to me" may give way to "not in my family." Adults who can't bear to think that their teens would violate the family values reinforce a system of denial.

Religion, sad to say, is sometimes at the root of denial, as well. Our faith mandates an abundance of life-enhancing values. But when guilt is the tool that "encourages" persons to live up to those standards, teens especially are not eager to admit that they haven't. Religion, improperly understood, can become a dangerous weapon of denial rather than a liberating means of grace.

Nobody is immune to this virus, but ignorance, fear, blame-placing, and denial put many at risk.

The Result

No matter how you get it you must remember that HIV is a chronic illness like cancer or multiple sclerosis. Some people can live with the HIV a long time and not show any symptoms. However, once you are infected, you have HIV until it moves through the stages to AIDS and you die.

A real concern among adults who work with young people who test HIV positive is that they try to deny what has happened. They may tell themselves that even though they tested positive, it will never turn into AIDS. Thus, they may not enter into an early treatment program that could greatly prolong their lives. Another common response is to simply deny the test results completely, thinking that they must be wrong. This frees this person to act as if he or she doesn't have the virus, and so he or she will probably still be active sexually.

Finding out you test positive is just like finding out that your cancerous lump is malignant. For most this is terrifying. Perhaps for the first time you are forced to deal with the reality of your own death and the possibility of life after death. While a person may live well for years before showing real symptoms, she or he will have to face what is now an incurable illness.

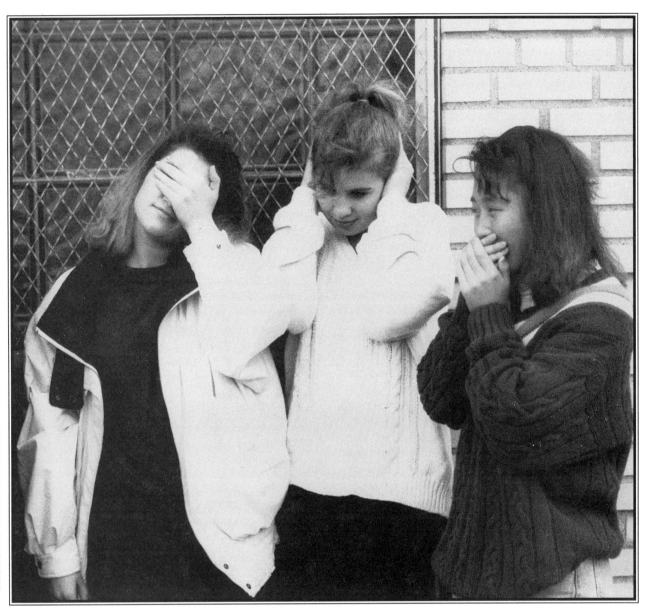

It seems easy to deny the fear by telling yourself that the news is not true. If you are in denial, then who will you be angry with? The person who gave you the virus? The person who gave him or her the virus? Yourself? Finally, how do you deal with your parents?

Parents

Rev. Howard Warren, a Presbyterian minister who heads the Pastoral Care area of the Damien Center, a center which ministers to those with HIV and their families, notes that many of the people he works with don't even tell their parents that they are HIV positive until their second or third visit to the hospital. There seems to be a fear of telling parents generally because they will have to deal with other issues such as their child being sexually active, homosexual, or an injection drug user.

AIDS Is in My Community

How many young people (18 and under) in your state are HIV positive? Do you know anyone your age who has the virus? In 1992 one of every thousand Indiana teenagers was HIV positive. What scares me is the vast majority (81% to 92%) don't know they are infected and so probably are still engaging in the risky behavior that endangered them and continues to endanger others. These young people don't think it can happen to them because they believe AIDS is something that happens in California or New York. Yet Indiana has one of the highest escalating rates of HIV in the U.S. in terms of the percentage increase. In fact the South and Midwest are showing the highest percentage increase in the country. Why do you think that is so?

The Bible

The Bible is silent on the subject of AIDS because it was unknown. The closest comparison we have is the biblical understanding of leprosy and the community's expectations about the treatment of persons with leprosy. The many laws about leprosy in **Leviticus 13 and 14** make it clear that anyone who might be infected was to admit it and get straight to a priest. If the person was truly sick, he or she had a flock of rules to observe, some of which seem rather cruel, such as being expelled from the community and having to cover his or her mouth and cry out "Unclean" when anyone approached.

If we tried to enforce similar laws, no one would want to admit publicly that he or she was infected with HIV, and that would make denial, delayed treatment, and protection of others even more difficult. In fact, we do try to enforce similar laws when we won't permit an HIV positive student to go to school or fire him or her from the job. The fear of rejection and worse is one big threat personally and a great ally to denial.

But we can gain from those biblical laws that denial was not a good idea. If treatment was possible, it was offered immediately for the good of the patient and the good of the community.

The Bible also offers us other passages that teach us better ways to relate to others than rejection. **Matthew 8:1-4** shows Jesus healing a man with leprosy. Jesus commends him to the priest, in accordance with the custom; but Jesus also touched him, a dramatic change from typical practice and a worthy model for us. When we refuse to reject others and then reach out, we work toward overcoming some of the dynamics of denial.

For Further Reflection

Lead a discussion about denial.

✤ What are the ways we deny what we don't want to believe?

✤ How do we hide things we don't want to know or don't want others to know?

✤ If your best friend tells you he or she is HIV positive, would you tell him or her to hide it from everybody? Why or why not? What might be the consequences of denying or hiding the truth? What might Jesus say to your friend?

✤ Since the virus is spread primarily through sexual activity and injection drug use, how do you think this affects young people who have to admit to their parents or other adults that they are or might be HIV positive?

Practice dealing with denial.

✎ Divide into pairs. Each person in the pair will "confess" to his or her partner that he or she has done something (he or she chooses) that could lead to HIV infection. The listener may ask questions only to draw out whatever information is necessary. When each partner has "confessed," have them answer these questions.

✤ How did you feel to admit to someone else that you had put yourself at risk?

✤ Compared to that feeling, what might your feelings be if you find out you are actually infected?

✤ Did you receive any assurance? What was the response of the person you told?

✤ What happened in the confession that made telling easier? harder? What did you learn from that?

✎ Now roleplay, in the same or different pairs, a situation in which each person is fairly certain that his or her partner needs to face up to a hard truth, but is unwilling to do so. For example, you tell your partner that you know his or her steady has been diagnosed with HIV and has asked you to break the news (another form of denial!). Then ask:

✤ How difficult (or easy) was it to break through a wall of denial? How did you feel?

✤ How did the denial make you feel?

✤ What successful techniques did you discover to help your partner face the truth? What didn't work?

✤ What did you learn?

Investigate the Scriptures.

✽ Read **Psalm 139**, noting especially verses 1-12. Use a commentary to help understand it. The psalm is one person's understanding of God's activity in his life. The psalmist affirms that there is nowhere he can go to be away from God. No matter where he is, God knows.

✤ What does this passage suggest about the possibility for denial?

✤ Can we really hide anything from God?

✤ How is God involved in your life? Is there any area where God is not actively involved? Do you believe that God is always with you?

✽ Look up **James 4:17; 5:12, 19-20** in the Bible and a commentary. These three statements are practical and direct in stating that we must address the truth and follow through on it.

✤ What do you think these passages suggest about denial? about getting to the truth?

✤ Can this biblical message help someone who is struggling with denial and reality regarding HIV infection and AIDS? Why do you think so?

Reverend Jeff Buck has been involved with youth ministry in the local church, district, and conference level, working particularly to help equip and motivate adults so that they can lead youth in faith and discipleship. Jeff presently serves as Associate Pastor at Castleton United Methodist Church in Indianapolis, Indiana. Jeff and his wife Julie have two daughters, Sarah and Anna.

The Church's Position on AIDS

by Jeff Buck

At First Glance

When AIDS was first recognized in the early 1980's, a number of religious organizations issued statements concerning the need for both education and research. Over the next few years ministries within the church grew, responding to the individual and community needs rather than to any denominational plan. Our whole culture during the mid-1980's really did not know how to deal with AIDS.

Is AIDS God's Judgment?

Shortly after the news broke concerning AIDS, there began a persuasive belief that AIDS was the direct judgment of God on homosexuals and intravenous drug users. This was believed because the first known cases were primarily within those groups. While some ministers and members of local congregations have accepted this belief, the church as a whole has not. In fact, the consensus of Roman Catholics, mainline Protestants, and Evangelicals is that AIDS is a disease (not a punishment) and each person deserves the care and love that Jesus would give her or him.

In the Church of the Brethren's paper, "A Call to Compassion" (1987); they say: "Whatever the causes that contribute to human illness, our Christian response to illness must be one of compassionate care. As followers of Jesus, and as members of the Church of the Brethren, we are called to be about the ministry of healing."[1] This Statement exemplifies the position of United Methodists, Presbyterians, Episcopalians, Lutherans, American Baptists, Roman Catholics, and nearly all other churches.

AIDS and Morality

However, the connection of AIDS and sexual immorality causes some real concerns. For example, note The Evangelical Free Church's Statement on AIDS (1986):

"Most victims of AIDS have been involved in a homosexual lifestyle which the Bible expressly condemns (**Lev. 18:22**) and which God will judge (**I Cor. 6:9-10**). There are also other victims of AIDS who have not been involved in homosexual activity but who are suffering the consequences of this presently incurable disease. . . . We reaffirm our responsibility as Christians to show Christian compassion to the victims of AIDS, both to those who are guilty of sin and those who are innocent victims. . . . We support the efforts to minister to victims of AIDS, we pray for progress in research efforts to combat the AIDS epidemic."[2]

Most churches struggle with the connection of AIDS and sexual immorality. The Southern Baptist Convention in 1987 spoke to the issue of AIDS: "We. . . go on record as believing that obedience to God's laws of chastity before marriage and faithfulness in marriage would be a major step toward curtailing the threat of AIDS; and be it further resolved, that we urge Christians to exhibit Christlike compassion in dealing with the hurting victims of AIDS and their families."[3]

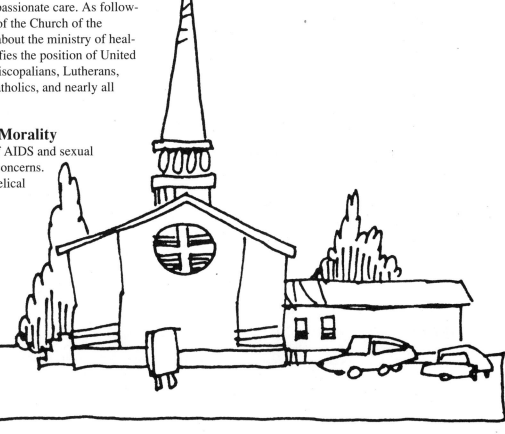

A Matter of Perspective

Frankly, back in the early 1980's, no one, including the church and the federal government, had any real idea of the global nature of AIDS. Do you see any change of outlook from the following reports? The United Methodist Church's first report was "AIDS and the Healing Ministry of the Church" (1988). It said: "According to the Gospel of **Luke (4:16-21)**, Jesus identified himself and his ministry with that of the servant Lord: the one who Isaiah tells us was sent to bring good tidings to the afflicted; to bring hope to the brokenhearted; to proclaim liberty to the captives; to comfort all who mourn; to give them the oil of gladness, and the mantle of praise instead of a faint spirit (**Isaiah 61:1-3**). . . . Diseases spring from complex conditions, factors, and choices. It is not helpful to speak of diseases in inflammatory terms like 'punishment for sin.' The Gospel challenges us to respond with compassion that seeks to enable the physical and spiritual wholeness God intends in the lives of all persons affected by Acquired Immune Deficiency Syndrome (AIDS)."[4]

Note the change to a more global awareness in "The Church and the Global HIV/AIDS Epidemic," a resolution adopted by the 1992 General Conference of The United Methodist Church: "The United Methodist Church will work cooperatively with colleague churches in every region in response to the global HIV/AIDS epidemic which is affecting the health and well-being of individuals and communities worldwide. . . . The New Testament presents a Jesus who reached out and healed those who came to him, including those who were despised and rejected because of their illnesses and afflictions. Jesus' identification with those who suffer was made clear in his admonition to his disciples, that 'whatsoever you do to the least of these you do also unto me' (**Matt. 25:40**). His great commission to his followers to go and do as he has done is a mandate to the church for full involvement and compassionate response."[5]

While there is some uneasiness concerning the primary ways AIDS is spread, the consensus of the church can be summed up in Cardinal Joseph Bernadin's (Roman Catholic) Pastoral Statement on AIDS (1986) (in responding to the belief AIDS is God's judgment): "It is important that AIDS be seen as a human disease that deserves that same care and compassion as any other disease."[6]

What Are Churches Doing?

Most denominations have an AIDS network of some kind. This network links individuals and ministries who work with persons with AIDS and their families. The United Methodist Church has a number of resources that are available for churches and for pastors to help minister to persons with AIDS as well as special resources for those with AIDS. Each annual conference has a committee or task force on AIDS. Contact them or your own judicatory body for more information.

For Further Reflection

Use these questions as discussion starters.

✤ What is your denomination's official stance on AIDS? Does your local congregation know it and assent to it? What parts of the official posture are problematic for your own congregation? Why? What is the area of greatest agreement?

✤ What is your personal response to AIDS? Do you think AIDS is an example of God's judgment? Why or why not?

✤ Some denominations affirm that the gospel calls us to offer compassionate ministry to persons with and affected by AIDS, but decry the use or distribution of condoms if that action could in any way be seen as affirming an immoral lifestyle or encouraging immoral behavior. What do you think of that? Why?

✤ Since AIDS is mainly spread through sexual activity and injection drug use, do you think AIDS is a consequence of sinful behavior? What does your denomination say?

✤ Does your denomination recognize the difference between the disease and persons who are ill?

✤ How do we minister to those with AIDS?

Study the Scripture.

✱ Read **John 9:1-41**, the story of a man born blind. The Pharisees and Jesus debate about whether the man sinned and who has the power to heal and to forgive sin. Particularly note the responses of Jesus.

✤ What happened? Who are the main characters and how do they behave?

✤ What does this passage say about illness and sin? about the religious response to illness?

Notes:
[1] J. Gordon Melton, *The Churches Speak on: AIDS,* (Detroit: Gale Research Inc., 1989) p. 75.
[2] Ibid., p. 81.
[3] Ibid., p. 130.
[4] Ibid., p. 148.
[5] From *The Book of Resolutions,* 1992. © 1992 by The United Methodist Publishing House. Used by permission.
[6] Melton, p. 3.

Rev. Jeff Buck has been involved with youth ministry in the local church, district, and conference level working particularly to help equip and motivate adults so that they can lead youth in faith and discipleship. Jeff presently serves as Associate Pastor at Castleton United Methodist Church in Indianapolis, Indiana. Jeff and his wife Julie have two daughters, Sarah and Anna.

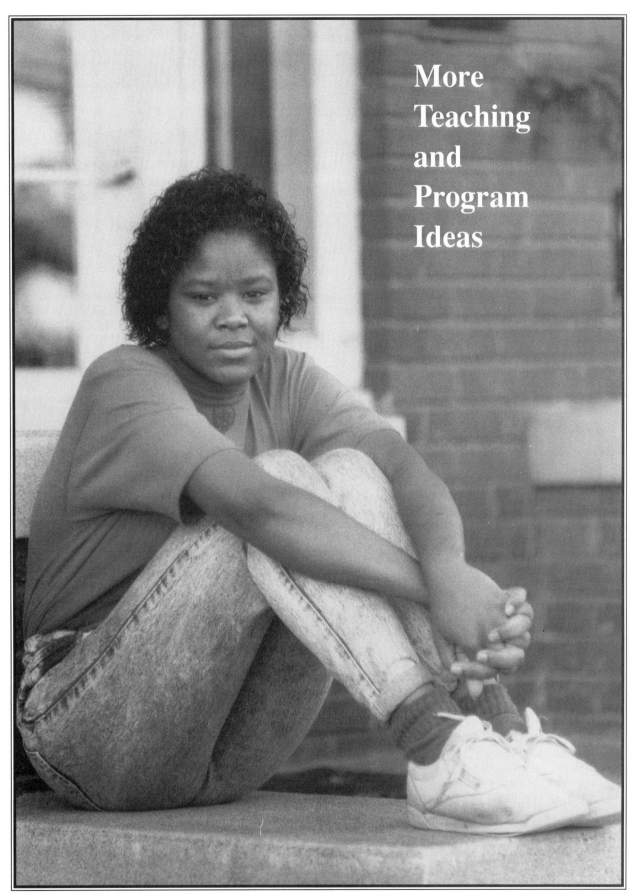

**More
Teaching
and
Program
Ideas**

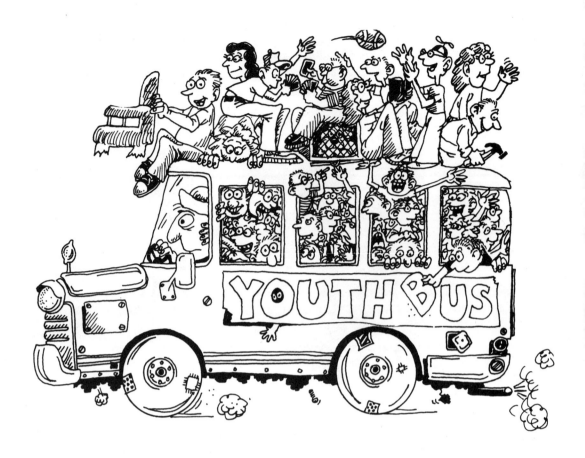

Guidelines for Talking About AIDS With Your Youth Group

1. Develop a willingness to talk about this subject in public. It may just take "psyching yourself up" to do it.

2. Make these points every chance you get:
➤ AIDS is fatal and there is no cure.
➤ The virus is spread by the exchange of body fluids (blood, semen, vaginal secretions, conceivably saliva) from one person to the mucous membranes at body openings of another person.
➤ You can catch and give AIDS because of what you do. The main ways that most teens will be exposed to AIDS is through unprotected sexual intercourse and IV drug use (including steroid use). The virus can be spread when sharing a tattoo needle or piercing ears!
➤ AIDS is a virus that does not discriminate—anyone can catch it. Although some persons are in higher risk categories than others, no one is safe if he or she practices risky behavior.
➤ The only 100% safe sex is no sex.

➤ A monogamous relationship, including marriage, is no protection from HIV/AIDS if one or both of the partners is already infected or engages in other risky behavior, like IV drug use.
➤ A relationship in which sexual intercourse is involved deserves sexual monogamy and marital fidelity.
➤ If a teen thinks that he or she may be infected, the teen should get tested. Teens should be as concerned about passing this deadly virus to another person as they are about getting it.
➤ Once someone has the virus, it is useless to dwell upon how it was contracted. Don't blame the person with AIDS; support and love that person.

3. Talk freely about ways other than sexual intercourse to express intimacy in a relationship. Help the youth know how to reject effectively any kind of pressure to participate in undesired sex acts.

4. Describe the proper use of condoms, lubricants, nonoxynl-9, and so on. Better still, arrange demonstrations. Some of your youth are or will become sexually active, and they need to know these things.

Discussing "Touchy" Subjects

If you're into guidelines, here are a few more to help you know how to broach touchy subjects with teens. These hints may help you be more approachable and more sensitive to the needs of your youth:

➤ Always try to give straight answers.
➤ Don't "come down" on a youth by being judgmental or demeaning.
➤ Don't be unrealistic.
➤ Don't take advantage of a situation or prey on the vulnerability of the youth in order to make a point.
➤ Maintain confidentiality. Decide right now whether your commitment is to a youth or to his or her parents. If it is to the youth, then you should encourage the teen to speak to his or her parents about the issue; you should not take it upon yourself to report to the parents unless it is a matter in which the youth is in imminent danger of physical harm.

If your commitment is to the parents, you should let the youth know before confiding in you. If she or he goes ahead with the issue, then you know that the youth wants the information to be communicated to the parent but may not be able to do that directly.

✎ If a youth approaches you wanting to talk at an inconvenient time, schedule the earliest possible time to meet the youth. Don't put it off because there is a good chance that the youth has already put off the conversation until it is almost at a crisis stage.

Program and Resource Ideas

✎ Acquire some of the resources listed on pages 94-95 and make them available to your youth in some discrete reading area within the church.
✎ Consider setting up a lending library (without check-out cards for anonymity reasons) with books and resources about AIDS and other touchy subjects. Make sure Magic Johnson's book is in your library.
✎ Make up some wallet-sized cards with the hotline numbers listed on pages 96 and following. Also include local hotlines and the telephone numbers of yourself, the pastor, and others in the congregation who could be helpful in time of crisis.

If you are on a church staff or are considering having calling cards printed for your youth ministry, print this hotline information on the back.

✎ Contact your denominational headquarters about programs like "Face to Face" who would be willing to send representatives to come to your church and tell their story. Don't limit this to just the youth. Parents and the congregation at-large should be invited to an adult session (which probably would go better if kept separate from the youth session).

"Face to Face" is an educational program sponsored by Northern Virginia AIDS Ministry (NOVAM). Parents have a preview of the program and youth spend time with a health educator. Student volunteers help spread the word on HIV/AIDS to other teens. Contact NOVAM at 413 Duke Street, Alexandria, VA 22314 (703) 739-2437.

✎ Sponsor the NAMES (AIDS Memorial) Quilt in your community. The 1992 quilt displayed in Washington, D.C. contained approximately 20,000 panels. The address and phone number are NAMES Project Foundation, 2362 Market Street, San Francisco, CA 94114 (415) 863-5511.

✎ PWA memorial bracelets are now available to help to raise the consciousness level of the public—especially of teens. Why not? It worked for the MIA/POWs.

All money raised goes toward providing emergency funding for people with AIDS and their families. These bracelets cost $10 and bear the name, age, and date of death of people who have died of AIDS. Students who can't afford a bracelet can receive one free in exchange for an original 300-word composition about AIDS. Call (213) 933-3662.

✎ Are there people in your church who have AIDS or whose loved ones are infected? There may be enough people in your church with this concern to form a support group. Make sure any youth find support even if it is simply one-on-one support from you.

✎ Help your youth learn how to treat people who have AIDS. Some suggestions from Magic Johnson's book include: don't avoid them; don't be afraid to touch; don't isolate them; cry and laugh with them; call before you visit; share a meal; share holidays; send cards to say "I care"; help with shopping; offer to help answer letters or phone calls that your friend may be having difficulty dealing with. What others can your youth come up with?

✎ If there are a number of younger teens in your church, consider inviting **Kids on the Block** to come do a program about AIDS or about dealing with PWAs. **Kids on the Block** is a national organization with chapters in many cities and towns.

The "kids" are actually large puppets that are manipulated by adults who are highly skilled in the ancient Japanese art of "Bunraku," shadow puppetry.

These are excellent plays and the organization assures the quality of each of its "kids" teams. Call 1-800-368-KIDS to locate the nearest **Kids on the Block** team.

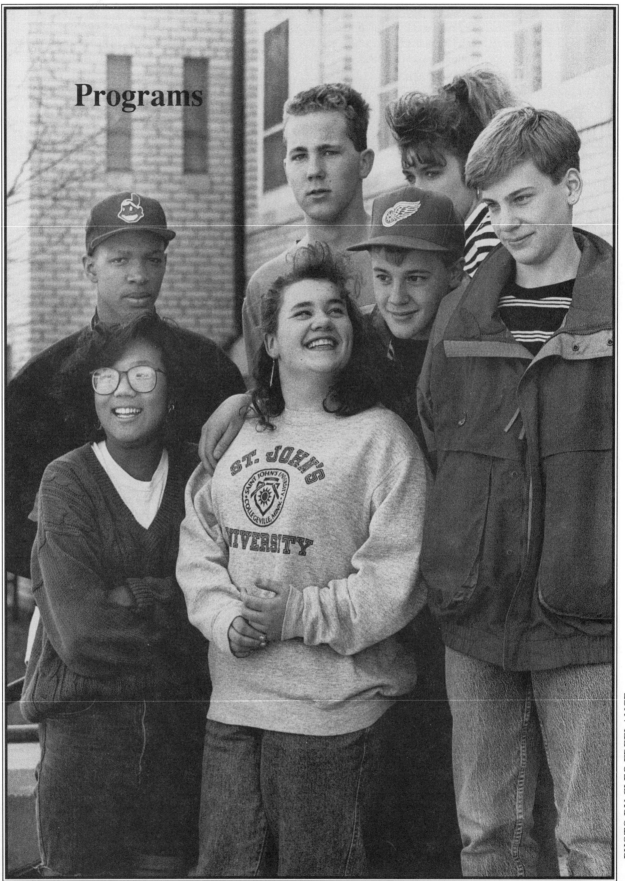

Programs

PHOTO BY CLEO FREELANCE

God and AIDS

by Diana L. Hynson

PURPOSE: *to help youth begin to think biblically and theologically about AIDS, recognizing that God is a God of grace and justice.*

An Abundance of Issues

The subject of AIDS conjures up numerous issues, both from a physical and social dimension and from the biblical and theological dimension. AIDS is a frightening, often loathsome subject. For many the jury is still out on how persons with AIDS should be regarded at work, at school, at church, and at home.

The most obvious physical and social issues are sexuality and sex, the treatment of one's body, rejection, illness and disease, and death. Persons in the church and community have responded corporately and individually in many ways, sometimes touchingly positive and other times unbearably negative.

The Bible offers a wealth of guidance about how we as Christians can and should view life and death and all matters in between. Understanding what the Bible says (and recognizing how we make our own interpretations) makes a world of difference in how we understand and respond to persons with AIDS and their families.

The most obvious biblical and theological issues that come to mind are discipleship and accountability, creation in God's image, steadfast love, compassion, hospitality, and death and resurrection. Over and through all those issues stand God's grace and justice.

This program will help you look at where God is when we confront AIDS as an illness and in its very human dimensions.

✎ Have on hand a Bible for each person, several Bible dictionaries and topical concordances, markers and newsprint or chalk and chalkboard, paper and pencils.

Imagine God

Our images of God greatly influence how we make meanings of our circumstances. To use two simplistic examples, if our image of God is of a kindly, "cosmic grandpa," we will interpret life events assuming that God wants good things for us and has the power to give them to us. Or, if we regard God as a judgmental, "wicked stepparent" figure, we will interpret life events assuming that God is not concerned with the good that we do, but only with our mistakes, for which we can and will be punished.

✎ Appoint one teen as scribe to record the answers of the others in the group. Brainstorm in two or three minutes all the words or phrases they can think of for God. Give the scribe a chance to add to the list.

✎ After listing the images, talk about which ones seem positive and which are negative. Note where the most images fall. (If most of the teens have a generally negative view of God, you have a lot of work to do!)

✎ Be prepared to add these images if they do not come up: steadfast love, compassionate, just, gracious, and savior.

✎ Discuss how the teens think and feel about God, especially how they perceive a relationship between God and themselves.

✎ Younger teens may have trouble making this connection, but invite the group to mention any instances when they could see how their image of God had (or has) an influence on how they interpreted a noteworthy event in their lives. Be prepared with an example of your own.

Can You Confirm the Image?

We all have images of God, but we don't always consciously know where those images came from. We hope they come from the Bible, but we inherit images or impressions from our parents and others, too. Since we closely tie in our concept of God with Father, we often find that what we think about God is curiously akin to our experience with one or more significant adults in our lives.

One image in particular is important for the teens to research: God's *steadfast love*. Simply stated, God's steadfast love is both the essence of grace (unmerited and unconditional love) and of forgiving accountability. In other words, God calls us all to an intimate relationship with God in which we are expected to uphold a faithful obedience to God's will. If we fail or fall short, God will correct or reprove us, but never fails to love us with an all-encompassing, forgiving love.

Many Scriptures refer to steadfast love, especially in the Psalms, but **Psalm 51** reveals it well. In this psalm of David, David freely admits his sin and repents, acknowledging God's justification to punish him. David also affirms God's power to forgive and God's "abundant mercy" and "steadfast love." He has every expectation that God will "restore the joy of salvation."

✎ Distribute the Bibles and other Bible research tools and divide the group into several teams. Mix older and younger youth in the groups. Either assign or have teams choose an even share of the images, words, or phrases of God from their brainstorming session.

✎ To make their research more fun, ask them to imagine that they are the church task force responsible for naming their new congregation. The church as a whole has decided to name the church something that reflects their concept of God, and the task force is to come to a congregational meeting with suggestions. Have them use their Bibles and research books to look up the images so that they have a fuller understanding of who God is and what that identity or image means in terms of a personal relationship. Ask all groups to look at **Psalm 51**.

✎ When groups are finished, bring them together to report their findings and recommendations. When all groups have reported, everyone should have several ways (perhaps new ways) to think about God.

Confront the Human Issues Theologically

Summarize briefly some of the key issues about AIDS from the social and physical perspective: the treatment of our bodies, sexuality and sex, illness and disease, stigmas and rejection, and death. Then mention briefly some biblical and theological responses to those issues: discipleship and accountability, creation in God's image, compassion, hospitality, death and resurrection, and grace with justice.

These lists of key issues and theological concepts do not neatly correspond. Rather, they are woven together into the complicated fabric of our human understanding of AIDS. Even if in different words, your images of God should suggest or reflect the theological issues.

✎ Divide the group into age level teams of three persons. Give each team a copy of the cases and ask them to select one or more to discuss. Ask them also to consider the questions that follow.

✎ When teams have had about ten minutes to talk about their case, come together and report your findings.

1. Jordan is on the wrestling team at your school. He was using steroids to pump himself up, shared an infected needle, and now is HIV positive. Since he is so newly infected, he looks and feels fine—physically. Emotionally, he's a wreck. He is turning to the coach and his buddies on the wrestling team for support, but he is turned away outright or "politely" given a lame excuse for why his friends don't want to be near him.

✤ What would be your immediate response as one of Jordan's friends?
✤ What do you think about his rejection? Is it a gracious and fair gesture from others?
✤ How do you think God would want you to respond? What image(s) of God come to mind that help you decide how you could feel, think, and behave?

2. Lillian is fifteen and her world is coming apart. She found out in the same lab report that she is pregnant and HIV positive. Chances are high that the baby will be infected, too. Since her boyfriend tested positive also, they are arguing about who gave the virus to whom, since both had been sexually active before. Her boyfriend is not interested in using condoms, although she did ask him once to use them. Lillian is trying to figure out if she should tell anyone else, who to tell, and how to break the news. Her boyfriend is just busy being angry.

✤ What is your immediate response to Lillian? to her boyfriend?
✤ What do you think about her situation? about what she should do?
✤ What do you think about the way Lillian and her boyfriend regard their bodies? Why?
✤ How do you think God would want you to respond? What image(s) of God come to mind that help you decide how you would or should feel, think, and behave?

3. Nineteen-year-old Conrad is a bundle of conflicting emotions. He has been struggling to sort out his own sexual identity. Conrad is well acquainted with the facts about AIDS and AIDS prevention. He has abstained from risky sexual behavior and confined his activity to hand-holding and kissing. When he found out his partner was HIV positive, he was tested too, just to be sure, at a clinic in a nearby small town. He tested negative, but a nurse muttered, "Too, bad. Would have served you right" and called him a nasty name.

✤ What is your immediate response to Conrad? to the nurse?
✤ What do you think about the issue of sex and sexuality in this context? Why?
✤ What is your image of grace and justice in this context?
✤ How do you think God would want you to respond? What image(s) of God come to mind that help you decide how you would or should feel, think, and behave?

4. LaReesa's brother died recently from complications of AIDS. Neither LaReesa nor her family ever commented publicly on how he contracted the disease, but she is aware that there has been considerable gossip and speculation (without any evidence) about his sexual orientation, possible drug use, and past friends—both male and female. While the family is receiving visitors before the funeral, LaReesa sees several of her brother's friends who never visited while he was sick. One of them says to her, "This is for the best. Now he's with God."

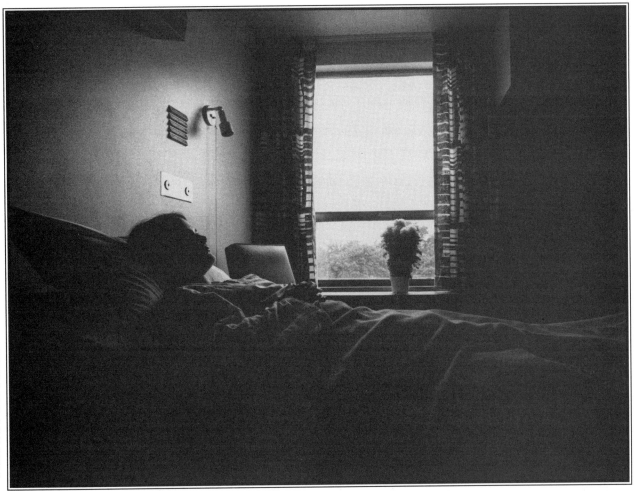

PHOTO BY JIM WHITMER

✤ What is your immediate response to LaReesa's situation? to her brother's situation?

✤ What do you think about the visitors at the viewing? about their comment to LaReesa?

✤ What is your concept of death?

✤ How do you think God would want you to respond? What image(s) of God come to mind that help you decide how you would or should feel, think, and behave?

5. Nikko tried injection drugs once, on a dare, when he was sixteen. Now he is twenty-seven; weighs a fraction of his normal weight; and is nearly consumed with Kaposi's Sarcoma, a form of cancer associated with AIDS patients. He has nasty-looking lesions all over his face and chest and most of his hair is gone. Nikko has been in the hospital this time for eight days and has had one visitor: his mother.

✤ What is your immediate response to Nikko and to his situation? about his mother?

✤ What do you think about compassion and hospitality in this context?

✤ How do you think God would want you to respond? What image(s) of God come to mind that help you decide how you would or should feel, think, and behave?

✎ When all small groups have talked about their cases, bring the whole group together. Ask them to report the highlights of their conversations, being sure to point out how their concept of God influenced what they thought and felt about each situation. Ask which Scripture they studied had an impact on the discussion. Report also on any new insights, changes in assumptions, and altered preconceptions.

Close With Prayer

Ask the group to gather in a circle and offer prayers for those whose lives are affected by AIDS.

Diana L. Hynson is an editor with The United Methodist Publishing House and has written for or contributed to several United Methodist publications.

Could Someone Like Me Really Get AIDS?

by Elizabeth Bower

PURPOSE: *to help youth sort out their feelings of fear about getting AIDS and to help them measure their own risk factor.*

Younger youth are concerned about their developing bodies and fear any diseases or situations that would make them different. Older youth are concerned with how the threat of AIDS affects their maturing sexuality. Both groups struggle with feelings from "It could never happen to me" to "I can't trust anyone."

Take an AIDS Inventory

AIDS is a disease that will lead to death. AIDS stands for Acquired Immunodeficiency Syndrome, and it is caused by the Human Immunodeficiency Virus (HIV). Because AIDS is one of the most serious health problems in the Unites States, it is important to talk with one another about what you know about the disease, how you can get AIDS, and how you can make some choices that will lower your risk of getting AIDS.

✎ Make a copy of the following statements for each youth or write them on a chalkboard. Ask each person to mark each statement true (T), false (F), or rumor (R) according to what they have read, have heard, or have been taught.

_____ 1. Everyone can get AIDS.

_____ 2. The only way you can get AIDS is by having sex with someone who has AIDS or the AIDS virus.

_____ 3. You can be infected with AIDS by sharing drug needles with an infected person.

_____ 4. Babies of women who have been infected with the AIDS virus may be born with the infection because it can be transmitted from the mother to the baby before or during birth.

_____ 5. You can get AIDS through everyday contact with people at school, work, church, the swimming pool, or the supermarket.

_____ 6. AIDS can be transmitted by insects.

_____ 7. You won't get AIDS by kissing a person with AIDS.

_____ 8. You won't get AIDS by coming in contact with the sweat, saliva, tears, or urine of a person with AIDS.

_____ 9. You may get AIDS from a blood transfusion if the blood is infected with the AIDS virus.

_____ 10. You can get AIDS from using clothes, the telephone, a toilet seat, dishes, or eating utensils used by a person with AIDS.

_____ 11. You can get AIDS in a Cardiopulmonary Resuscitation class by using a resuscitation doll if a person with AIDS also practices with the doll.

_____ 12. You can always tell if a person has AIDS or the AIDS virus.

_____ 13. Male, female, heterosexual, bisexual, or homosexual persons are all at risk of getting AIDS.

_____ 14. The best preventive measure for teens against sexually transmitted AIDS is avoiding all sexual contact.

_____ 15. AIDS can be medically cured.

✎ Discuss the statements above as a group. You may want to invite a person who is knowledgeable on the subject of AIDS to be present to answer questions, or you may want to provide up-to-date printed materials that would help separate fact from rumor. Point out that concern about AIDS is appropriate but that the fear of getting AIDS may be magnified by rumors and lessened by factual knowledge.

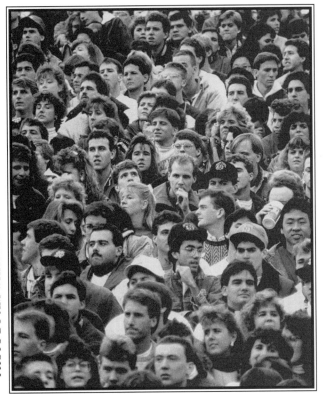

PHOTO BY JIM WHITMER

✎ Before the program, write the following behaviors on typing paper, one behavior for each sheet of paper. The risk category follows the behavior; do not indicate it on the paper. Tape to the wall three signs indicating the degree of risk: low, moderate, and high. Distribute the papers to the students and ask them to tape the papers on the wall, placing them in the appropriate risk category.

   a) a person who has unprotected sex with a person who has AIDS (high; that person is taking a BIG chance, not only for an STD, but for pregnancy, too)
   b) a person who has protected sex with another person (moderate or low, depending on how careful they are. Condoms break and can be misused.)
   c) a person who has surgery and has a blood transfusion (low, since the beginning of blood testing)
   d) a married couple who are sexually faithful to each other (low or completely safe, if they have not and do not engage in other at-risk behaviors)
   e) a health care professional (doctor, dentist, nurse, and so forth) (low to moderate; surgeons may be at greater risk, since it is not unusual to nick a finger and contact contaminated blood from a patient during surgery)
   f) a person who shoots drugs (low, if the works are sterile, but a very stupid thing to do!)
   g) a person in a hospital or nursing home (low)
   h) a first grader who sits next to a child with AIDS (low)

   i) a person who uses another person's needle to shoot drugs (high; that person has a death wish)
   j) a police officer who comes in contact with a bleeding accident victim (low, if the victim is not HIV positive. The risk could be higher if the officer contacts contaminated blood through a cut or other wound.

✎ Since extenuating circumstances can change the risk categories, take time to find out and discuss why teens have responded as they have. Discuss any myths or erroneous thinking, and explain the facts.

What Does Our Faith Say About AIDS?

Ask: What does our faith say to us about AIDS? Have the group read together **1 Corinthians 6:18-20** and answer the following questions.
✤ What does it mean to say the body is a "temple of the Holy Spirit"?
✤ How would living out that statement mean we were safer from AIDS? (The major ways in which AIDS is spread are casual sex and drug use, both violations of the body as a temple.)

Options for Older Teens

✎ Look again at the true-false statements above.
   1. Go around the group and take turns changing the false statements into true statements. (For example: Statement 12 would read "You cannot always tell if a person has AIDS or the AIDS virus by his or her physical appearance.")
   2. Go around again and personalize each statement. (For example: "I cannot tell if a person has AIDS or the AIDS virus by his or her physical appearance.")
   3. Go around again and make the personalized statement plus a statement of conclusion. (For example: Conclusion: "I will not assume that a healthy appearance means a person does not have AIDS or the AIDS virus or that a frail and sickly person must have AIDS.")

✎ Invite each person to make a personal commitment to:
➤ helping others understand facts about AIDS and
➤ living a life that is free from behavior that is high-risk for AIDS.

(At the time of this writing, the answers to the statements according to the CDC information, October 1992, are as follows: 1. T 2. F 3. T 4. T 5. F 6. F 7. T 8. T 9. T 10. F 11. F 12. F 13. T 14. T 15. F)

Elizabeth Brower has written for Directions in Faith for The United Methodist Publishing House. Liz has a Master of Arts in Religious Education from Union Theological Seminary and has worked as a Director of Christian Education in local churches.

How Do I Relate to People With AIDS?

by Grant Hagiya

PURPOSE: *to help youth sort out how they feel about people with AIDS and to encourage them to relate to people with AIDS in the spirit of God's love and care for all persons.*

Preparation

✎ Before you lead other people through the session, read through the whole program. Do the forced choice exercise, "I'm OK; You're . . ." and try to sort out how you feel about people with AIDS.

✎ For the activity "I'm OK; You're . . ." set up the room so that participants can move around easily. You will also need to decide on a process for dividing the youth into small groups. Have available a Bible for each person.

I'm OK; You're . . .

This activity is a forced choice exercise, which means that the teens will have to choose how they would respond to a particular set of circumstances.

Post the Signs.

On one side of the room, post a sign that reads, "I don't want anything to do with him or her." On the opposite side of the room, post a sign that reads "I have compassion for him or her; I will get involved." In the middle of the room, post a sign that says "Neutral."

Explain the movement.

After hearing each description, the teens are to move to one side of the room or the other depending on their reaction to the person you describe.

Record who stands where.

As the youth express their feelings about each of the people you describe, write down the number of youth standing on each side and in the middle of the room. The tally will help refresh your memory as you lead the reflection.

Have the teens keep track of their answers.

Ask the youth to keep track of their thoughts and feelings during the activity so that they can talk about them later.

Explain the setting.

Begin by saying: "Your church has developed a program in which volunteers call on people in a local hospital. You are part of a team of volunteers. Each time you visit the hospital, a nurse reads descriptions of the people individuals in your group may visit. After each person is described, you will choose whether or not to visit him or her."

Read the following descriptions of people.

➤ a drug addict with a long criminal record, who contracted AIDS by using contaminated needles

➤ a classmate who tried injection drugs only once on a dare

➤ a young gay man who contracted AIDS from one of his sexual partners

➤ a fourteen-year-old boy who has hemophilia and contracted AIDS through a blood transfusion

➤ a one-week-old baby whose mother had AIDS and transmitted the disease to her child at birth; the mother contracted AIDS from a sexual partner

➤ a senior girl in your school who has the reputation of being "easy"

➤ a senior guy in your school who has the reputation of being a real "hunk"

➤ your cousin who contracted AIDS from a blood transfusion during surgery performed a number of years ago

➤ your best friend who has been diagnosed with AIDS, the source of which is unknown

Reflect on the Choice Exercise

Have the youth divide into small groups of three to five people. Invite the groups to talk about their thoughts and feelings during the activity "I'm OK; You're . . ." and to discuss the following questions:

✤ How do you feel about the fact that so many different types of people have contracted AIDS under so many different circumstances?

✤ Did you feel compassion for some but not for others? Why?

✤ On what was your compassion based?

✤ What do you know about AIDS and its transmission?

✤ Would having more information change the way you relate to a person with AIDS?

✤ Do you know anyone who has AIDS? Does knowing someone personally make a difference in how you feel?

✤ Would you be willing to actually minister to and serve a person with AIDS? Why or why not?

For the Leader

Dealing with a fatal disease is difficult; AIDS also carries with it a social stigma. Persons with AIDS have to deal with other people's judgment, blame, curiosity, anger, fear, and revulsion. Many persons with AIDS are rejected by their families, friends, work associates, churches, and even themselves. Some are rejected

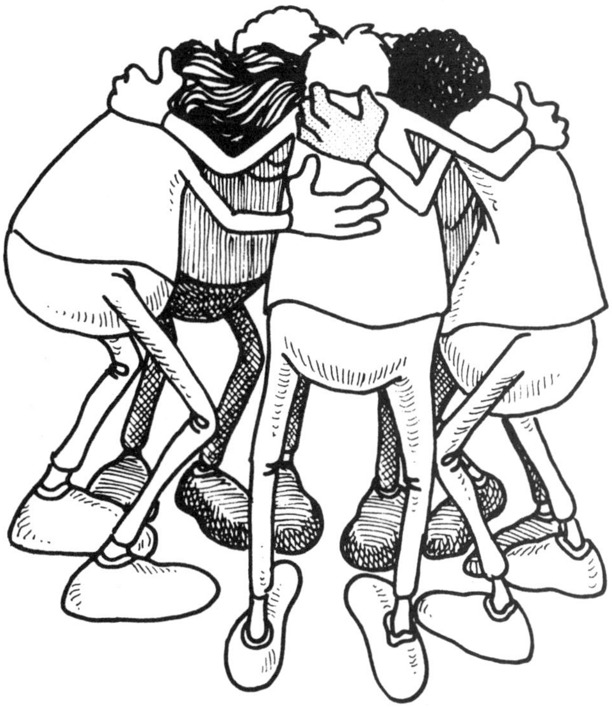

because the people around them, including some church people, think that AIDS is a homosexual disease and/or a deserved punishment. Some persons with AIDS whose families and friends love and support them discover that no one is willing to kiss them, touch them, or get too close to them. They often report feeling like lepers must have felt in biblical times (see **Leviticus 13,** especially verses 45-46).

On the other hand, family members, friends, classmates, or colleagues of a person with AIDS also find it difficult to deal with feelings about the disease. In some cases, they have to cope with the surprise or shock of learning that a person they care about has been engaged in at-risk behavior. Family members wonder *Why me?* and feel disappointment and grief knowing that the person with AIDS is seriously ill and will die in the not-too-distant future. Family members who are well and the person with AIDS go through a similar grief process. While they cope with their own feelings, they may find it difficult to support the person who is sick. Friends, classmates, colleagues of people with AIDS may want to be supportive but may fear being labeled homosexual. Others may be concerned that their homosexual orientation will be discovered.

As members of the youth group begin to sort out their feelings about AIDS, they may express some of the feelings that people face when a friend or family member has AIDS.

What we feel about AIDS and what we know are two different things. Give the youth plenty of time to express their feelings in this time together.

We're All OK With Jesus Christ

Divide the youth into four small groups and give each group one of the following sets of instructions:

❊ Read **Mark 1:40-45.**

Leprosy in biblical times was in many way like AIDS in our contemporary world. Leprosy was feared and regarded as repugnant. It had no cure. People thought that leprosy was contagious and spread by contact with people who were infected. Yet Jesus touched a man with leprosy.

Answer the following questions:

- Knowing that in Jesus' lifetime people considered leprosy to be deadly, how do you feel about Jesus' response to the leper?
- How do you think the leper felt when Jesus cared about him?

✤ In this Scripture, Jesus' touch was motivated by pity or compassion. Might compassion motivate you to touch a person with AIDS? What affect do you think your touch would have on him or her?

✳ Read **Hebrews 13:1-2.**

The Scripture reminds us of our obligation to hospitality and mutual love and suggests that strangers may be sent by God. We never know what blessings God may have in store for us.

Answer the following questions:

✤ What is true mutual love?
✤ What does *hospitality* mean? In biblical times, hospitality meant more than being neighborly. It involved unselfishly sharing possessions so that a guest would be treated kindly in every way.
✤ Do you feel obligated to show hospitality to others? Why? Why not?
✤ Do you think a person with AIDS could be an "angel" without your knowing it? Why? Why not?

✳ Read **Luke 10:25-37.**

The Scripture suggests that a person we reject (the Samaritan) could have a positive influence on us. Believing we are superior does not make us superior, nor does it free us from needing each other.

Answer the following questions:

✤ Who is your neighbor?
✤ Could a person whom you fear, dislike, or disregard do a kindness for you? Why? Why not?
✤ Do you think a person with AIDS should be despised as the Samaritan was? Why? Why not?
✤ Would you accept help from a person with AIDS? Why? Why not?

✎ When the groups have discussed their assigned Scripture passages, bring the groups together. Ask:
✤ What have you learned?
✤ In what ways has your thinking changed?
✤ How have your beliefs changed?

Now What?

In this session, the youth will have sorted out some of their feelings about AIDS and about people with AIDS. They will have realized that everyday people—their friends, neighbors, relatives—could be among those infected with the disease.

Brainstorm ways to relate to persons with AIDS

Invite members of the group to brainstorm and to make a list of ways they might want to relate to people with AIDS. The list may include ideas such as the following:
➤ to support the family of a person who has AIDS
➤ to support a classmate who has AIDS and to help

change negative attitudes toward him or her
➤ to inquire at a local hospital about holding or feeding babies who have AIDS
➤ to work with a state or local task force on AIDS to promote an AIDS awareness program at church or school.

Find ways to follow through

After the youth have listed several items, ask them to select one or two of the ideas they listed and to begin working on plans to follow through on them. Since relating directly with AIDS patients can be emotionally draining, be sure the youth and their parents are clear about what to expect and about what will be expected of them.

Optional Activities

✎ Invite someone with HIV/AIDS to speak to the group about his or her experience with and feelings about the disease. If you choose to ask a person with AIDS to speak to the group, be sure the teens are prepared (and their parents). They should think through some of their feelings about AIDS, discuss ways of making sure their guest feels welcome and comfortable, and decide the questions they want to ask. Some questions may be too personal or too judgmental and should not be asked. Before the session, give your guest a list of questions so that he or she can be prepared. Provide your guest with clear information about the occasion for the meeting, the audience, and the time.

Contact your state or community AIDS hotline for information about speakers. More infected teens are becoming peer counselors and are prepared to speak directly, frankly, and culturally to teens.

✎ Invite members of a state or community task force on AIDS to participate in a panel discussion. Help teens prepare for the discussion as they would for a guest speaker.

✎ Invite a pastor, doctor, nurse, social worker, and an elected official to participate in a panel discussion. The members of the panel should have worked with persons with HIV/AIDS and their families or with community groups or legislative bodies concerned with public policy that affects persons with HIV/AIDS and their families.

Grant Hagiya is Director of Urban Ministries and Assistant Professor of Religion and Society at the School of Theology at Claremont, California.

When AIDS Comes to School

by Mary E. Brown and Traci D. Patton

PURPOSE: *to help youth deal with the various dynamics of being in school with persons who are HIV positive or who have AIDS.*

Introduction

HIV, the virus that causes AIDS, has impacted our nation in many ways, including our school system. Transmission and prevention information is taught in science, health, or home economics classes. Rumors, jokes, and misinformation is shared in the locker rooms and hallways. And the virus itself is being transmitted in the back seats of teens' cars.

Teenagers are aware of HIV/AIDS, are concerned about it, and some have even changed their behavior because of it. But what is the relationship of HIV/AIDS to our teens' school life? Teens may be overwhelmed with information, unsure of what kind of response is appropriate. In some communities, emotion-charged debates are occurring as decisions are being made regarding curriculum or admission policies concerning an infected student. Most often these debates do not include the students themselves, so the students may lack an arena to discuss and process feelings regarding sexuality education or discrimination. This program will give teens a chance to explore their own feelings, and will introduce a process to better understand the feelings of others as well.

Advance Preparation

Gather newspaper and magazine articles that relate to HIV/AIDS. Investigate your own school board policy regarding HIV infected students and staff. See the resource section on pages 94-95.

AIDS at Your School

Post or display the newspaper and magazine articles that you gathered. As the youth enter, ask them to look over the resources. After you have welcomed everyone, ask them if they feel like they know a lot, some, or a little about HIV/AIDS. Encourage the teens to answer the following questions freely.

✤ How is AIDS presented in school (in which class is it taught, does the teacher feel comfortable teaching the subject, and so forth)?
✤ Do you know if there are any infected students at your school? any infected teachers?
✤ Do you know anyone who is infected?

Remind the students that most of us do know someone who is infected, but we just don't know it. The Centers for Disease Control estimates that one in every 250 peo-

ple is infected with HIV. Many people who are infected do not even know themselves that they are infected, because you can be HIV positive and look and feel healthy.

Safe Contact at School

✎ Ask the youth to divide into groups of 6-8 people. (This activity can be done in a large group if desired.) Give each small group a sheet of newsprint and a marker. Ask them to brainstorm the answers to the following questions. (Remember the rule of brainstorming: everything is written down without evaluation.)

✤ What activities at school could put you at risk of contracting HIV?
✤ What school activities are not risky?
✎ After five minutes, ask each small group to look over the list and evaluate the responses to be sure that everyone agrees with the risk described. Then ask each small group to present their list to the large group. In the large group, try to find consensus on risk levels. Clear up any misconceptions. Possible correct answers include:

Safe contact:
Restrooms, telephones, water fountains, desks, hand rails, doorknobs, pencil sharpeners, showers, sharing a locker, contact sports, being around someone who is infected, hugging, holding hands.

Unsafe Contact:
Contact with someone's blood, semen, or vaginal fluid; sexual contact; sharing needles or syringes.

Should Persons With HIV/AIDS Come to School?

✎ Tell the youth that there is a diversity of opinions regarding teaching about HIV/AIDS in the schools and allowing someone who is infected to attend school or work in a school. People base their opinions upon facts, fears, prejudices, values, and beliefs.
✎ In order to better understand the range of feelings that exist, use the following roleplay with your youth. Ask for volunteers or assign these roles to your teens. Give them a few minutes to read over their roles and to understand the situation. Make copies of the situation for each role player. Make nametags for each roleplayer with his or her name only.

The situation
Ryan is a small town that could be anywhere in the United States. The local school board is sponsoring a town meeting to discuss an issue that is on everyone's mind: AIDS in the school. The state Department of Education has required each local school system to adopt a policy concerning HIV education. The school board must

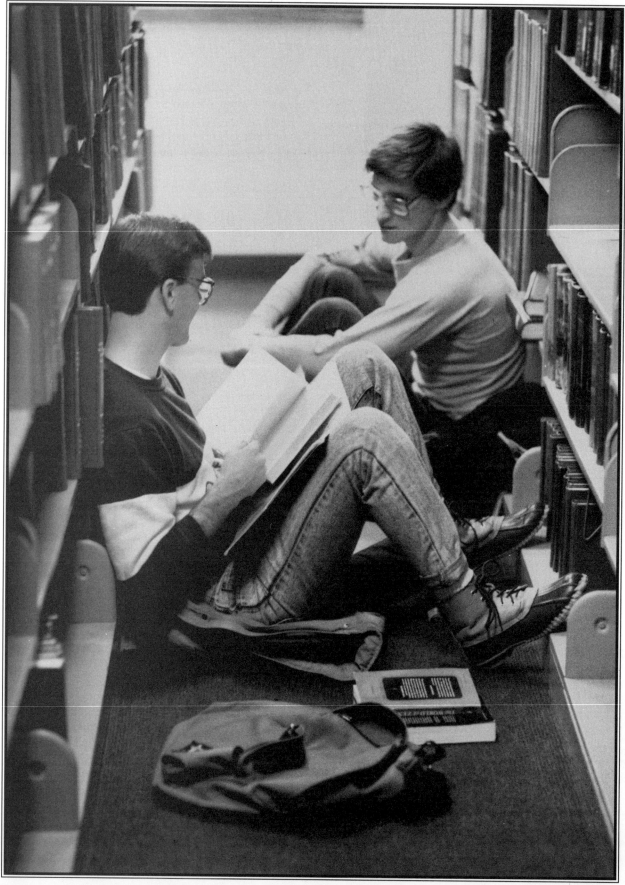

also adopt a policy regarding HIV-infected students and teachers. Ryan officials decided to open up the issue to a town meeting. Parents, students, and citizens of Ryan are present. The meeting is to be an open forum to investigate people's thoughts and fears.

The Participants

• Ms. Carol Johnson (played by an older teen or adult), is superintendent of schools and moderator of the meeting. Ms. Johnson's role is to keep people on the subject, and she does not express her own opinion. She makes sure that everyone has a chance to speak and that no one is judged or attacked for expressing an unpopular opinion. She might say: "Thank you for your opinion," or "Remember, we all have the right to speak."

• Tom Jackson, a teacher who has taught in Ryan for 15 years. Tom is active in his local church, is married, and has two preteens. He does not want the school board to allow someone who is infected to attend school or work there. He is concerned about the risk of providing first aid if someone is injured or of someone getting in a fight and biting someone else. He might say: "But what about protecting me and my rights," or "I don't want to be forced to take any chances at all."

• Cindy Wilson, a young woman in her twenties who has just moved back to Ryan. She lives with her parents. Cindy is HIV positive and is beginning to have health problems. She will likely be diagnosed with AIDS within the next six months. She is unable to work and wants to volunteer to teach about HIV/AIDS in the schools. Very few people know she is infected. She might say: "I contracted this virus when I was a teenager. Teens need to know the facts."

• Robert Novella, father of a 10-year-old child who recently died from complications of AIDS. The Novella family moved to Ryan after Todd's death. No one else in the family is infected. He might say: "Todd enjoyed his friends and school so much. I'm glad that he wasn't isolated from his peers."

• Stacey Frazer, a concerned member of the community. She does not have her opinion formed, but she is cautious. She asks a lot of questions and does not have all her facts straight. She might say, "But I heard that the virus can be spread through saliva," or "We need to be sure to do the right thing."

• The other participants. Your role is to be yourself. Discuss the issues from your own opinions. Bring up issues that you and your friends are concerned about.

✎ After everyone has read his and her roles and understands the situation, ask the person playing Carol Johnson to begin the meeting and to open the floor for discussion. Continue for about 15-20 minutes. (It is very important that no one is judged or attacked for the opinions expressed.)

✤ After the time limit, ask everyone to stay in character and discuss how he or she would feel if the meeting had ended as your meeting had.

✤ Ask the teens to come out of character and ask: Did the group come to any decision? Was there consensus? Were people open to listening to each other?

✤ Ask each person if he or she learned anything. We each hold our own values, attitudes, and beliefs very dear. Sometimes it is hard to listen to people whose beliefs are different from our own. It can also be hard to understand why someone feels a certain way if we do not know that person well.

Where to Go From Here

Each of us needs to understand about HIV because it is very likely to touch our lives personally. The statistics show us that many of the people who develop AIDS contracted the virus when a teenager. The issue is relevant. What kind of response should we make to this epidemic? How can a teenager help? Brainstorm some possible responses and develop plans to follow through, especially for ways teens can be involved at school. Listed are a few possibilities:

✎ Learn more about HIV and be a source of facts for your friends and family. Call the National AIDS Hotline at 1-800-342-AIDS for information.

✎ Pray for people who are infected with HIV, their families and loved ones.

✎ If you know someone who is infected, be a friend to that person. Don't be afraid to talk about his or her HIV infection with him or her. He or she may also want to talk to you about God, death, and being afraid. Encourage your friend to take care of him or herself, and to take advantage of available community resources.

✎ Work with your school health or science teacher, guidance counselor, or other school personnel to establish a school support group for students who are HIV positive or who have AIDS. An added support group can be formed for students to help them say no to the at-risk behaviors that lead to infection. In time, the support groups can support and educate each other and other students. Even though the support group is at school, consider making prayer and Bible study a part of the support and nurture.

✎ Volunteer to help an AIDS service organization. Volunteers are needed to help in many ways, including answering hotline calls, being a buddy to someone who is sick, and providing peer education. Call the National AIDS Hotline at 1-800-342-AIDS for information about organizations in your area.

✎ Encourage the adults in your church to learn more about HIV/AIDS and opportunities for service.

✎ Don't put yourself at risk for HIV, and encourage your friends to also avoid risky behavior.

Mary Earheart Brown serves as Education Director for Nashville CARES, a community-based AIDS service organization. She graduated from the University of Kentucky with a degree in Family Studies. She is a member of Brookhaven Cumberland Presbyterian Church where she teaches Sunday School and directs the Childrens Choir.

Traci Denean Patton works as HIV Prevention Specialist for Nashville CARES, a community-based AIDS service organization. She graduated from Western Kentucky University with a degree in Public Relations. She is an active member of Lake Providence Baptist Church in Nashville, TN where she serves as a Youth Minister Associate.

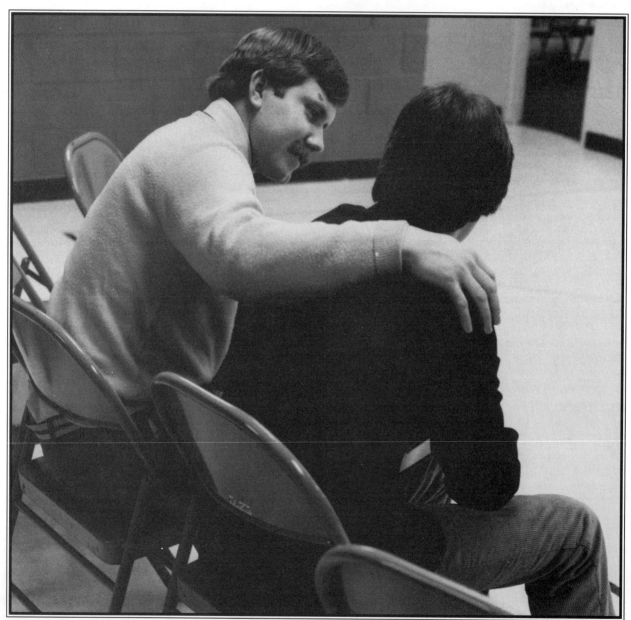

PHOTO BY JIM WHITMER

Parents Deal With AIDS

by Fritz and Etta Mae Mutti

PURPOSE: *to help parents whose children have HIV/AIDS cope with feelings and attitudes about the disease and about their children.*

Rethinking Our Assumptions

None of us want to see our children hurt or in pain. When our children are small, we kiss the hurt away or we sit and hold them for long hours until the fever breaks. We vicariously take on that pain ourselves, and the child feels safe and secure when he or she is in our arms.

How do we react if that child is an adult? The first impulse is to rush to him or her and again take that child in our arms and kiss away the hurt. Is the reaction different, though, when we discover the illness is AIDS? Probably. There may be that first fear that the disease is contagious and we must not kiss our child or allow our child to breathe or cough on us. Or there may be anger. How could our child do this to *us*? Didn't he or she know how to avoid getting AIDS and making *us* suffer? Of course, some did know how and others were unaware that unprotected sex or dirty needles would cause their illness or death. But that angry feeling is still in us. We did not (or do not) use drugs. Why is our child doing that? We were not (or are not) promiscuous. Why did our child choose that lifestyle? There are many, many feelings that overwhelm us when we first discover that we will probably outlive our child. The book "Love You Forever," written by Robert Munsch, offers a picture of life in which the child takes care of the mother when she is old and unable to take care of herself. With AIDS this usually doesn't happen.

Take Inventory of Your Feelings

✎ Write the letters "HIV/AIDS" down the side of a sheet of paper. Using the letters separately, try to think of a feeling you have had that begins with each of the letters.

As you review the words you have written, you will become aware of the wide range of feelings that come to each of us when tragedy strikes. You are not alone in having these feelings, and you are certainly not wrong in having them.

✎ Find a partner other than your spouse and compare lists. Discuss your answers to the following questions.

✦ How many feelings are similar? dissimilar?
✦ Did you feel justified or guilty about any of your feelings? Which ones? Do you know why?
✦ Did you or do you feel alone in those feelings? If your partner has expressed the same feelings, does that make you feel any different? If so, how?

Why Me? What Will Others Think?

Have you ever wondered why you are the one to whom this is happening? As you look around at your friends, it seems that their children are next to perfect. They marry persons you would want for your child. They give your friends beautiful grandchildren. Why isn't this happening to you? Are you being punished by God for something that you feel is not really your fault? How do you pray to a God with whom you are angry?

All these questions surely have been asked by you or some of your friends. What a comfort it is to turn to God at times of self-doubt and self-accusation. It takes a lot of *talking* with God finally to be convinced that you did nothing wrong. It also takes a lot of *listening* to God to be able to say, "I can handle this, no matter what happens, because I know God is going to be beside me."

One of the dilemmas we have as parents of children with AIDS is when and how much to tell our friends. It sometimes takes a long time to process the information privately and then to make the grief known to our friends and acquaintances.

✎ Make a list of ten of your closest friends. Consider the reactions you might receive from each of them, such as:
  ➤ Will immediately give you a hug
  ➤ Will cry with you
  ➤ Will listen and express sympathy
  ➤ Will show shock and ask how your child became infected
  ➤ Will listen then change the subject.

✎ Form pairs, if possible, of one person who has already talked to family and/or friends and one person who has not. Without mentioning any names (or make up names) of friends or family, jot down who you think would respond in what way. You are not limited to the suggested reactions listed above.

✎ After making your list, discuss with your partner any fears you have or have had. Talk about how to prepare yourself to disclose difficult information by anticipating reactions and your response to them.

When to Tell and When Not to Tell

Predicting the reactions of others will help you decide whether to talk to your friends or other family members and when the best time might be when you do decide. Although we kept our knowledge of our sons' illnesses hidden for a year and a half, one of the best things that happened to us was to let our friends know. The love and care with which they surrounded us gave us the support we needed. We received what it was not possible for us to give each other.

It is easy to keep the tragic truth hidden when your child is in good health, but the time comes when it will be obvious to everyone that something is seriously wrong. Perhaps this is the time you will choose to make it public.

✎ Keeping in mind your previous discussion, work in the same pairs to respond to these questions:
✤ Do you have any potential supporters? What clues make you think so?
✤ Have you thought through how to respond to unkind remarks (intended or not intended)?
✤ Do you know how you feel about your child? about AIDS? about the circumstances in which your child contracted HIV?
✤ If you disclose the news, will it help you? your spouse? your infected child?

✎ After taking stock, take turns practicing a situation in which you break the news to someone else. Decide who will play which role and try to anticipate the reaction of the one who learns and the response and approach of the one who is telling. After each of you has had a turn, talk about what went well, what didn't, what felt comforting, what didn't, and what those reflections suggest for a real situation in which you break the news to a friend or family member.

When Your Child Is Far From Home

Being seriously ill or facing death when you are many miles away from home can be an extremely lonely time. How can parents make the right decision about how much time to spend with their child?

When a child is close to you geographically, perhaps in the same town, it is easy to pop over with some home-cooked food or to call and offer to do some shopping for him. However, when parent and child live far apart, these visits cannot occur so often. Part of that is due to scheduling and part to finances. Airline tickets are expensive, so we must choose the times carefully when we make the trip. Should you visit every time your child is sick in bed or only when she is in the hospital? Should you insist that he come home when he is too sick to take care of himself or should you go live with him and take care of him for an extended time? Those are options we may explore and decisions we must make. How hard it is! At times we may feel that our child does not want us around and wants to be with her friends rather than us when she is sick. How *could* that child choose them over us when we are the ones that took care of her when she was a child and saw her through all those adolescent years? But, we must remember that we are dealing with an adult, not the child we took care of, and that adult child is now the decision maker regarding his own life.

As our child gets sicker and sicker and time seems to be running out for all of us, we want to cling longer and harder to her. We want to be there every moment of every day to make sure things are made easier for her, and dur-

ing that time our hope fades and we realize more and more how futile everything is. But, the child does not always feel that hopelessness; sometimes she is the one giving us courage and forcing us to take a second look at what is happening to her.

✎ Form groups of four and discuss one or more of the following situations. Try to think through: What would I do? What is my motivation? What are my priorities and how do I decide?

1. Your child has attempted suicide and is in the psychiatric ward of the hospital 800 miles away from you. You feel you should go, even though he or she has not come right out and asked you to come. However, your spouse is receiving an important award in two days and you want to be present.

2. Your child is in the hospital 1,000 miles from you with pneumonia. He has been there for several days awaiting the test results. He calls to tell you it is pneumocystis pneumonia, which is one of the opportunistic diseases common with AIDS. You were not even aware that he had tested positive for HIV. You have dinner guests arriving in 30 minutes.

3. The doctor has told your child that she has only three months to live. You have known for some time that she had AIDS, but your spouse had not been told. The child wants to come home for an extended time, but your spouse, when finding out, has lots of anger and denial.

Remembering Fred
Our son had been in bed at home for two weeks before going to the hospital where he had a three-week stay. He was so weak he could hardly make it from the bed to the chair without becoming completely exhausted. The doctor thought he would last only a few weeks and suggested we bring him home with us until his time was up. However, our son, Fred, wanted to tend to some important matters: he wanted to go to his friend's wedding, to his tenth high school class reunion, and to Alaska. He bought the tickets to Alaska, in spite of protests from us. Two days after leaving the hospital he went to his friend's wedding in a wheelchair (and even danced with the bride, in his wheelchair). Two weeks later he went to Alaska and spent fourteen days there, then he came home to his high school class reunion. People were amazed, but Fred saw nothing unusual about it. His courage and hope in the future renewed ours. We were able to feel that each time he had a serious illness, he would come back from it until one day there would be a cure for this dreaded disease and he would be one of the first to overcome the illness. It was that hope and that fiery spirit of our son's that helped us through the dark days. As long as there is life, there is hope.

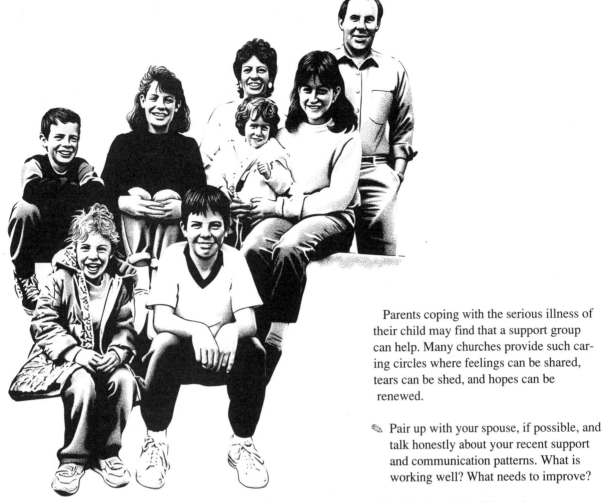

AIDS and the Rest of the Family

Coping with the serious illness of a family member is very difficult for siblings and sometimes devastating to marriages.

It is not easy to explain to other family members that one child needs you more than another one does. Siblings feel they are missing out on the love that should be theirs because there is no time left over for them.

Husbands can feel the same way when the wife becomes consumed by the attention needed from the person with AIDS. Many marriages end in divorce because of this stress. It is imperative that husband and wife keep the communication lines open and keep a constant check on how each other is doing.

There is a tendency to neglect communication, partly because of physical weariness. A tired body leads to a tired mind and neglected relationships: maybe tomorrow we will talk with our spouse and make sure he or she knows we still care. Maybe tomorrow night we will cook dinner for our spouse, maybe tomorrow we will take our spouse out for an evening of relaxation, maybe tomorrow. Sometimes that tomorrow never comes and the spouse decides it is time to go another direction and find a place where he or she doesn't have to face the illness of a child or the constant haggard and worried look of the spouse. Tend to your marriage.

Parents coping with the serious illness of their child may find that a support group can help. Many churches provide such caring circles where feelings can be shared, tears can be shed, and hopes can be renewed.

✎ Pair up with your spouse, if possible, and talk honestly about your recent support and communication patterns. What is working well? What needs to improve?

The Role of the Church

Where does the church fit into all of this? Isn't that where we should be finding all that hope and courage? Yes, the church is alive and functioning for persons living with AIDS and for their parents. The church is at its best when reaching out with love and care to those who are ill. The church reflects Christ when it offers love and compassion. Within the Christian community, there are people just aching to care for someone who needs them, someone to ask for help, someone to love.

✎ List fifteen things the church could do for you or for your child.
✎ Put a dollar sign by the things that would cost more than $25.00, a "1" by the service if it could be done by one person, or a "C" if it would take the help of several members of the congregation.
✎ Review the list and discuss the items that could be viable options for support from and with your congregation. Check with your Council on Ministries to help you follow through.

Fritz and Etta Mae Mutti are the parents of three sons. They lost two of these sons to AIDS. Fritz is a bishop in The United Methodist Church. Etta Mae's career has been as a church secretary.

Leader's Guides

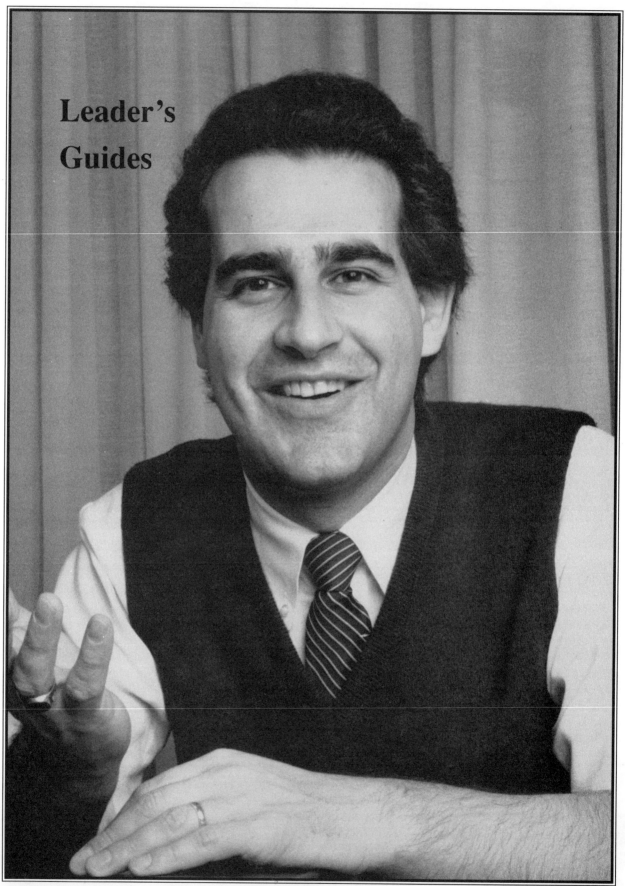

PHOTO BY JIM WHITMER

Leader's Guide for *Spread the Word*

by Laurel Schneider

Introduction

SPREAD THE WORD is a video for teenagers about teenagers and AIDS. It touches on a number of important issues confronting everyone dealing with the epidemic—issues such as grief, denial, fear, love, and commitment to change. *Spread the Word* contains interviews with young HIV positive persons, excerpts from AIDS-related theater performed by teenagers, and conversation among groups of teenagers involved in the third AIDS Memorial Quilt display in Washington, DC.

The video is available from Cokesbury for sale for $49.95. *Spread the Word* may also be available from Ecu-Film for a rental fee of $25.00.

To order from Cokesbury call toll free: 1-800-672-1789. Order no. FF2-339168.

To rent from EcuFilm call 1-800-251-4091 and ask for the video by name.

Prepare Yourself

This Leader's Guide should help you to focus group discussion before and after viewing the film. Because discussion of AIDS and the content of the film may well trigger intense emotional reactions and elicit deeply held attitudes and prejudices, you should prepare yourself by reviewing these materials carefully. AIDS has been a particularly difficult epidemic for most churches to address. As the following discussion will suggest, this film and your leadership present an opportunity for teenagers to re-evaluate Christian compassion and to confront Jesus' challenge to his followers regarding outcasts.

It will be important for you as a discussion leader to spend some time examining your own beliefs and fears about AIDS, to educate yourself about the disease itself, and to begin to distinguish between the medical phenomenon of AIDS and your beliefs and prejudices about the persons who suffer from AIDS.

The film *Spread the Word* offers important factual information about AIDS; but more importantly it puts human faces on the sufferers of AIDS, both those teenagers with the disease and those who have lost important people to the disease. As a leader, you are in a special position to help interpret and make real the love of Jesus as Jesus himself made it real: in unpopular and controversial places where he showed that healing love was the avenue of God's grace. You can help to facilitate the important teachings offered by the youth in the film to the youth in your group. As one visitor from Pennsylvania to the AIDS Memorial Quilt says, "kids can help to teach each other a lot easier."

"Never Thinking How the Victim Must Feel": What Is AIDS?

Early in *Spread the Word* a rap group sings about the cruel treatment AIDS sufferers receive in our society, "never once thinking how the victim must feel." AIDS in America is much more than a disease. Reactions to HIV, to AIDS, and to persons with AIDS have been intense and deeply emotional. Often theology and religious beliefs have played an integral role in the way that persons with AIDS have been perceived and treated. Why is this the case?

There are quite a few reasons why it is important for youth and adults to understand the disease called AIDS in a religious context. Some of these reasons will be addressed in this section. Others may arise out of your group discussions.

What do AIDS and persons with AIDS have to do with the church and your faith in God? How you respond personally to this question will deeply affect the kind of spiritual guidance you can offer to teenagers. Because the appearance of the disease in North America has elicited such extreme public reactions from church-based groups, it has been easy to confuse the disease called AIDS with persons afflicted with it.

As a medical phenomenon, HIV and the affliction of AIDS is no different than other difficult, deadly diseases in need of cures. It is most easily transmitted through unprotected sexual contact, and so it is similar to herpes or gonorrhea. It is difficult to treat and is deadly, so it is similar to cancer, leukemia, and heart disease. It can be transmitted through the blood, and so it is similar to malaria or hepatitis.

Unlike these other diseases, however, AIDS has sparked enormous popular controversy in our society. It has had churches up in arms. It has had citizen groups in protests of all kinds. It has had its victims kicked out of grammar and high schools; refused jobs, medical treatment, and insurance; shunned from neighborhoods; and despised on television. Why is the same not done to the victims of other serious and deadly ailments?

The answer is, of course, complicated. In part, it has to do with the fear that accompanies any new disease prior to the discovery of a cure or vaccine. People dying without a clear cause and without a clear cure makes everyone nervous. But even still, AIDS seems to be different. Enough medical knowledge about the disease was gathered so that the general public *should* have calmed down several years ago.

The knowledge of how to avoid contracting AIDS has been around now for a while. Cancer is equally deadly, herpes is sexually transmitted, hepatitis is passed around through drug use, and *The New York Times* reported in October 1992 that health workers are much more afraid of contracting tuberculosis from patients than AIDS.

Even the common cold is much more infectious. But still a diagnosis of HIV is reason enough for fear and for persecution of persons with the disease. One student travelling to the AIDS Memorial Quilt in Washington DC says, "Why? Why the continued uproar about AIDS and the poor treatment of its victims? What is a Christian understanding of this situation and what is a Christian response to it?"

"AIDS Is the Cruelest 4-Letter Word I Know": Denial and Rejection

Spread the Word introduces you to three persons who contracted the HIV as teenagers. Tara and Duane both got the disease through unprotected sex with infected partners. Ryan White, who appears on the video in his last interview, contracted AIDS from infected blood transfusions before blood donations were tested for the virus. All of them faced rejection, fear, and prejudice because of their illness. Ryan was refused entrance to his school. Duane tells of losing his closest friends when he became ill, and Tara says that she did not tell anyone at school out of fear of rejection.

Most of the dramatic skits deal either with the rejection of persons with AIDS or denial of the disease altogether. As one male student from the California School of the Deaf says, "a lot of people are avoiding the subject of AIDS. They make insults about AIDS and jokes about AIDS . . . I used to be the same way. I used to insult those people . . . and at school we would pick on them. Now I realize that AIDS isn't funny."

To begin with, it is very important to remember that public reactions to the presence of HIV and AIDS have had very little to do with the disease itself. Reactions to the AIDS epidemic have had much more to do with the persons who suffer from the disease. One doctor has suggested that AIDS is a modern symbolic equivalent of leprosy, and its victims are the same as the proverbial lepers of the Bible.[1]

"Then Christ Came and Knelt Beside My Bedside": People With AIDS and the Church

Because the disease appeared in North America most prominently in the gay male population first, AIDS has become cemented in the public mind as a gay disease. Gradually however, as more and more straight people contract it, AIDS is perceived as a disease affecting a wider population, particularly persons who received blood transfusions before the AIDS virus was identified, intravenous drug users, and persons who engage in unprotected sex with multiple partners.

Persons with AIDS report that the very first question people ask them is how they got the disease. "My cousin died at age twenty-four of a brain tumor," says nineteen-year-old Maryann Johanson, who has lived with AIDS for two years now. "Nobody ever asked him how he got it, as though he had done something wrong."[2] When basketball star Magic Johnson first revealed that he had AIDS, he had also to reveal how he may have gotten the disease. He disclosed the fact that he had led a sexually promiscuous lifestyle, engaging in unprotected sex with many women.[3] "Straight guys like Magic talk about all their sex with women to prove they're not gay," suggests one gay man dying of AIDS. "Somehow in this society, if you're gay, people think you deserve AIDS, like it's God's punishment or something."[4]

The idea that AIDS is a form of divine punishment for homosexuality, for sexual promiscuity, or for drug addiction is a pervasive and insidious myth that persists in many Christian communities and churches. What does it say about the Christian God to suggest that this terrible disease is a punishment? First of all, it says that Jesus was wrong about the God of love who *cares for* even "the least of these." In **Matthew 25:31-46**, Jesus challenges the disciples to distinguish between the righteous and the unrighteous on the basis of their love for the outcasts, the weak, the sick, the poor, and the unpopular. Jesus tells his followers that at the time of judgment, the unrighteous will ask, "Lord, when was it that we saw you hungry or thirsty or a stranger or naked or sick or in prison, and did not take care of you?" Jesus' answer is simple and direct. "Truly I tell you, just as you did not do it to one of the least of these, you did not do it to me." (**Matthew 25:44-45**) Jesus devoted his ministry to the message of acceptance of the despised, making the outrageous claim that they would be the first to enter the kingdom of heaven.

In the play *Threads, Needles and Patches*, excerpted in the film, a young character with AIDS describes his moment of death: "I spent the last few days of my physical existence wrestling with God. . . . Then Christ came, knelt beside my bedside, and asked me softly to take his hand. Then, I looked into his eyes, and I realized I had seen him before, throughout all my life, in each of you." The Christian challenge to youth and adults is to learn to seek Jesus where we might otherwise least expect him.

It may be helpful for you to review some of the stories of Jesus and the lepers who came to be healed, especially **Luke 5:12-13**. Lepers were the social outcasts of Jesus' time, and they suffered many of the same prejudices as persons with AIDS in our time. These people were considered untouchable, yet Jesus touched them and loved them.

What does this tell us about how Jesus would have responded to the AIDS epidemic? Jesus gives us another strong clue in his story of the good Samaritan. Look again at the story in **Luke 10:29-37**. An unidentified man lies bleeding and bruised by the roadside. Three persons happen along—a priest, a Levite, and a Samaritan. Only the Samaritan stops to help.

What is important about this story in this context is that Jesus tells us *absolutely nothing* about the man lying half dead on the road. He tells us much more about the three who pass by. But Jesus clearly does not think that it is at all relevant to tell us a thing about the man on the road, except that he is hurt. Was he good? Was he bad? Was he gay? Why did the robbers pick him? Was he a drug user? Did he sleep around? Was he a pillar of his community? A drifter? A saint? A politician? The point is, *Jesus doesn't care.*

Jesus is not interested in the character of the dying man. But he is very interested in the character of the men who passed by. A man is bleeding, hurt, and dying; and Jesus doesn't ask, "how did he get it?" He asks, "who will help him?" Those who preached love and justice pass by the dying man. This is the real sin. The love and acceptance of the Samaritan, Jesus tells us, is the love and acceptance of God.

"We Can Say, 'I Love You' in a Lot of Ways"

AIDS is a disease that is affecting everyone. Some of us are on the road, and people are lying dying at our feet. Jesus is interested in *our* character, how we will respond. AIDS is also a disease that affects some of our most basic beliefs about relationships, sex, and responsibility. Gay men, possibly the most despised group of people in America, are facing enormous loss, grief, and tragedy. They also constitute the group working hardest to educate and protect the rest of the society, even those who wish them dead.

Interestingly enough, the largest group other than gay men that is working to educate the public about AIDS is made up of lesbians, the *lowest* AIDS risk population in America. Gay men are educating themselves about safe sex; they are seeking communities that can help them establish and maintain monogamous relationships in a world that is hostile; and the incidence of AIDS in the gay population is dropping faster than in any other population. The people are not the issue.

Not a Punishment, but a Disease

AIDS is not a punishment for certain kinds of behavior. If it were, then pill poppers would get AIDS as much as intravenous drug users, but they don't. If it were, then businessmen who cheat on their wives but use condoms would get AIDS, but they don't. If it were, then lesbians would get AIDS as much as gay men, and gay men who practice safe sex would get AIDS, but they don't.

The point is, AIDS is a terrible disease that kills innocent people and terrible people; it kills people who have converted to Christianity and people who haven't. No person with AIDS deserves it. And no teenager should enter adulthood ignorant of the risks. It is important for youth to have support and counsel in their church communities that takes them seriously. Abstinence is the best method of avoiding AIDS, and the one the church recommends, but remember that Jesus does not condemn those who are not abstinent.

Entering a Religious Discussion

A religious discussion of AIDS with youth needs to take seriously the options that youth themselves are facing in their lives. Care of oneself and one's neighbor also means sexual responsibility and caution regarding drugs. What is missing in our lives that sex and drugs somehow seem to fill?

Reflecting on this question may help your group to establish the underlying theme of Jesus' ministry of love. Love yourself enough to take care of yourself. Love your future life partner (and possibly children) enough to wait. Also love your neighbor enough to accept him or her as God's beloved child, even if he or she has AIDS.

Samaritans were the despised people in Jesus' time, and it is a Samaritan who reached out to help when those who had more power, influence, and acceptance in society passed by. A common bumper sticker reads, "Fight AIDS, not people with AIDS." Jesus would probably have it on his car.

Questions for Discussion

✤ The film is entitled *Spread the Word*. What does this phrase mean to you now? One girl tells us that "kids can teach kids a lot easier." Do you agree? What are specific examples in your life that would be "spreading the word?"

✤ AIDS in America is much more than a disease. Reactions to HIV, to AIDS, and to persons with AIDS have been intense and deeply emotional. Often churches and religious beliefs have played an integral role in the way that persons with AIDS have been perceived and treated. Why is this the case?

❖ What do AIDS and persons with AIDS have to do with the church and your faith in God?

❖ The idea that AIDS is a form of divine punishment for homosexuality, for sexual promiscuity, or for drug addiction is a pervasive and insidious myth that persists in many Christian communities and churches. What does it say about the Christian God to suggest that this terrible disease is a punishment?

❖ Lepers were the social outcasts of Jesus' time, and they suffered many of the same prejudices as persons with AIDS in our time. (See **Luke 5:12-13**.) These people were considered untouchable, yet Jesus touched them and loved them. What does this tell us about how Jesus would have responded to the AIDS epidemic?

❖ The story of the good Samaritan is another good example (**Luke 10:29-37**). An unidentified man lies bleeding and bruised by the roadside. Three persons happen along; a priest, a Levite, and a Samaritan. Only the Samaritan stops to help. A man is bleeding, hurt, and dying; and Jesus doesn't ask, "how did he get it?" He asks, "who will help him?" Why doesn't Jesus care about the identity of the man or what lifestyle he lives?

❖ Is AIDS a gay disease? What groups have worked hardest to educate the public about AIDS and the risks of AIDS? What are the highest risk groups? What are the lowest risk groups?

❖ What does care for yourself and for your neighbor mean in the age of AIDS? Who are you protecting when you abstain from sex or practice safer sex?

❖ Put in your own words one thing you think Jesus might say to you and your friends about AIDS.

[1] Dr. Nancy Tatum, Department of Ethics and Medicine, Vanderbilt University, 1992.
[2] Personal correspondence, 1992.
[3] See the general news coverage of Earvin "Magic" Johnson's revelation of infection with the AIDS virus throughout the Fall of 1991.
[4] Anonymous, October, 1992.

Laurel Schneider is currently pursuing her doctorate in theology at Vanderbilt University in Nashville, Tennessee. A native of Massachusetts, she received her M. Div. at Harvard and served a United Church of Christ parish in Cambridge, MA. She has contributed to several publications (most recently *Soundings: An Interdisciplinary Journal*) on issues of theology and society.

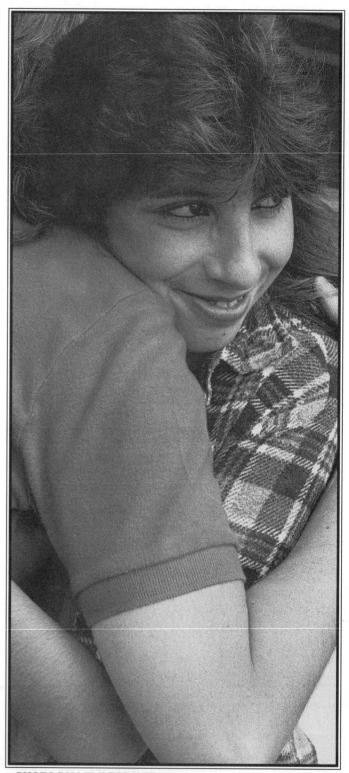

PHOTO BY MIMI FORSYTH

Wake Up, World
A Review of
What You Can Do to Avoid AIDS

by Andrew Cornell

It's Time to Wake Up!

It's time to learn that Human Immunodeficiency Virus (HIV) and Acquired Immunodeficiency Syndrome (AIDS) are out there. Yes, even if you are one of the finest Christians around, if you are not careful, you can get it!

Earvin "Magic" Johnson, in his book *What You Can Do to Avoid AIDS,* is telling it exactly as it is. AIDS can happen to anyone. In simple, clear, and at times very descriptive language, the book gives you basic information—and more. Magic answers all the questions you can imagine and even some you probably would never dream of asking.

Educating Your Church

Magic covers the AIDS epidemic from a medical and social perspective, and he gives solid background for beginning a discussion. (See the Leader's Guide on the next two pages.) The book does mention that if you have any questions concerning HIV or AIDS, one person to talk to could be your minister. Some ministers are leading their churches in the fight against AIDS. Unfortunately too many churches and ministers are still avoiding this subject. In the long run this avoidance will hurt people who will not learn or discuss the Christian perspective on the AIDS virus.

Magic says, "We are all God's creatures and we all deserve love and compassion." Doesn't that include someone with HIV or AIDS? What happens to you and your faith when you discover a friend or loved one has acquired the disease? Magic clearly states that you might feel helpless. But try a simple phone call or visit to tell your friend, "If you need anything, just call." This will make him or her feel comfortable and loved, and it will make you feel better. What do you think Christ would do in that situation?

More Than Basketball

You might ask yourself, "Why should I read this book? I will never get AIDS." Or you might think, "I'll read it, I'm a big fan of Magic and the Lakers." Think again. It is important to read it as though Magic is just another person, not a basketball superstar. Although the Los Angeles Lakers made Magic famous, he only mentions the Lakers once. He clearly shows that AIDS is a more important issue than basketball and that anyone, including super athletes, can acquire HIV.

This book includes personal stories from people who have acquired HIV and AIDS. These are everyday people: young, old, black, white, male, female, heterosexual, and homosexual, who tell about their lives before and after they acquired the AIDS virus. The stories back up everything Magic tells you throughout the book. The final section of the book includes phone numbers of AIDS hotlines and other related hotlines from each state, Canada, Puerto Rico, and the Virgin Islands. Most are 800 numbers, so they won't cost you anything.

It's hard to find a major weakness in the book. Some passages do seem to drag on with facts. But, while it is tragic to see anyone with HIV/AIDS, this book might sound the wake-up call the world has been waiting for. Since Magic made his surprise announcement, more and more people are being cautious with their sex lives. In addition, more people are getting tested—a crucial step toward prolonging and saving lives.

One final note: pray for Magic and others who have the virus. And pray for the men and women who are trying to find the right formula to cure AIDS. Hopefully one day the cure for HIV and AIDS will be discovered.

What You Can do to Avoid Aids is available in many local bookstores or can be purchased through the publisher: Times Books, New York, NY 10022; ISBN 0-8129-2063-5, for about $4.00.

Andrew Cornell is a graduate of High Point College with a BA in English Communications. Currently he is a US-2 working with publicity at the Scarritt-Bennett Center in Nashville, Tennessee.

Lite Up a Life: A Study Guide for "Magic" Johnson's Book,
What You Can Do to Avoid AIDS

by Diana L. Hynson

Beginning a Study

✎ *Some parents would rather talk to their children themselves about sex and other at-risk behavior.* With the level of AIDS education in the schools, it may not be unusual to discover that teens know more than their parents. In any case, notify parents and other interested adults and keep them informed. Give your home phone number so the parents can call you if they have any questions.

✎ *Emphasize more what "Magic" says rather than who he is.* Be careful of the extremes of harsh judgement and of rationalizing away personal responsibility. Magic is a well-known public figure who has contracted a deadly disease. He is insistent that he is not a hero; just a person trying to bring some good from a personal tragedy. It is important not to glorify Magic or the disease.

✎ *Talk about follow-through.* After using Magic's book and the rest of this resource, teens will have a better understanding of HIV and AIDS. Talk about ways to follow through with how each youth can take what he or she has learned to educate others, take the necessary precautions, assist those with the disease, and continue to have faith that one day AIDS will just be a memory.

✎ *Take time for prayer and reflection.* At the end of each session it is important that everyone take time for personal reflection. Finally, take time to pray for persons with HIV/AIDS, their families and friends, the researchers who are searching for a cure, and the churches for their continued support.

✎ *Page numbering in this Guide.* The page numbers refer to *What You Can Do to Avoid AIDS*, unless otherwise noted.

What is HIV/AIDS and Terminology (Chapter 1)

✎ Use the other programs and articles with HIV/AIDS inventories (see pages 7 and 36 of this resource) in conjunction with the book to help teens test what they know. Review the difference between HIV and AIDS (page 12).

✎ Review the basics in anatomy and anatomical terms (pages 16-19), terms related to the disease (pages 12-15), and to drug use (pages 20-21).
(There are basic line drawings on page 19.) Play a game like *Jeopardy* to review terms.

✎ Take inventory of the myths and questions (pages 24-35). Use a quiz bowl format.

✎ Clarify the facts about testing (pages 36-44). Be sure to offer support to any teen who feels he or she needs to be tested and especially to any teen who has tested positive. See the section "When Someone Comes to You" (pages 57-64 in this resource) for more insight into pastoral care issues. The personal anecdote on pages 45-47 gives one person's perspective on coping with discovery of HIV infection. There are others in the section "Teaching Articles" (see especially pages 10-14 and 18-20 in this resource).

Sexual Responsibility (Chapters 2, 3, 4)

Being sexually responsible is still a touchy subject to discuss in the church. The official stances and statements of several denominations are noted in the introduction and are on pages 27 and 28 in this resource.

✎ Separate into gender groups, each with a same gender adult leader. Look at pages 48-53 about understanding sexual feelings. Discuss the teen's feelings and experience. Do not judge. Answer questions and help teens express their feelings. If the teens want to share their conversations with members of the opposite sex, have a group session.

✎ Emphasize sexual abstinence before marriage as a viable and best choice. Point out and read pages 58-62, which offer teens' perceptions about abstinence. The article on page 9 in this resource, "Saying No to Sex," offers good reasons to abstain and some coping techniques to help teens say no.
Discuss ways to help build a support system among teens and with adults for teens who want to stand firm in the midst of negative pressure to have sex.

✎ Not all teens resist or want to resist, and they engage in sexual activity. It is imperative that they know how to protect themselves and their partners. Use the "big four" questions on pages 54-58 and information on pages 64-66 about talking to a partner to engage in dialogue about personal responsibility and sexual activity.

✎ Invite a sex education instructor or health care professional to talk to the teens about safer sex, including information about condoms and other methods of birth control.

✎ Use the "15 lousy excuses" on pages 87-92 to discuss safer sex. Move from there to the box on pages 77-79 (a personal "war" story about buying condoms) to talk about feelings about buying and using condoms. Point out the "Food for thought" comment about having sex and using birth control.

✎ Being married is no safeguard against HIV/AIDS. Use the personal story on pages 101-105 to talk about some consequences of unprotected sex.

✎ Define and describe other STDs (chapter 4) and how they are transmitted and treated. Encourage teens to seek medical attention if they have any reason to believe they are infected with an STD.

AIDS and Drinking/Drugs (Chapter 5)

✎ Emphasize the first sentence of Chapter 5 about the power to choose. Discuss with teens how they feel about their choices, what their choices are, and how they make choices.

✎ Use the personal story in the box on pages 128-130 to talk about the consequences of a variety of at-risk behaviors. Bill speaks about leaving a legacy; a way to reclaim some worth for his life after making many poor choices.

✤ Ask: What choices did Bill make? What do you think of those choices? Have you been faced with the same kinds of choices?

✤ Talk about what kind of legacy Bill is leaving. Ask: Is leaving a legacy a reason to engage in risky behavior? Does it justify making poor choices? What kind of legacy do you want to leave? Why?

✎ See also pages 16-17 in this resource on AIDS and drugs.

Dealing Personally With AIDS (Chapter 6)

The church should be a major support for someone who has the virus and for his or her family and friends. Make sure that teens understand this and that the pastor is prepared to be in conversation with them. See also the section, "When Someone Comes to You."

✎ The information on "What should I do if I have HIV?" (pages 131-137) and "What should I do if I have HIV and get pregnant?" (pages 137-139) should also be shared with all adult leaders and friends of teens. Set up some roleplays to help teens get a feel of

what it would be like to confront the discovery of HIV/AIDS. Consider these scenes and use the following questions to discuss the roleplay.

✤ Your best friend tells you that he or she has just been diagnosed with HIV. What do you do? Has your faith been affected? Has your friendship been affected by this news?

✤ Your cousin (or other relative) tells you he or she is infected with HIV and asks you to promise not to tell anyone about this. What do you do? What would you say to convince your relative how important it is to tell others?

✤ One of your school friends is becoming very sick with AIDS complications and you know he or she would appreciate some support. What can you do?

✎ Turn to the segment on how to help a person with HIV/AIDS on pages 139-145, especially the list beginning on page 141. Brainstorm with the teens ways to implement any of the suggestions that are appropriate for their current circumstances. Their actions and interest will vary depending on whether they know (and how well they know) anyone who is infected.

Choose several of the suggestions (or admonitions) about helping and practice how to follow through. If visitation is one choice, roleplay a visit so that teens can anticipate what will happen. Practice confronting difficult feelings with love and without judgment.

Runaways and Homelessness (Chapter 7)

✎ Use the suggestions and information to acquaint the teens with the available resources for teens who are on the streets. If you have a homeless or runaway teen, be sure to cultivate trust and to take an interest. As soon as you can, call on professional sources of help for that teen.

✎ The more mature and better informed teens may be able and willing to offer some peer counselling and support services at neighborhood teen shelters. Check with local resource persons.

Diana L. Hynson is an editor with the Department of Youth Publications at The United Methodist Pubishing House in Nashville, TN. Diana has edited and contributed to several youth publications.

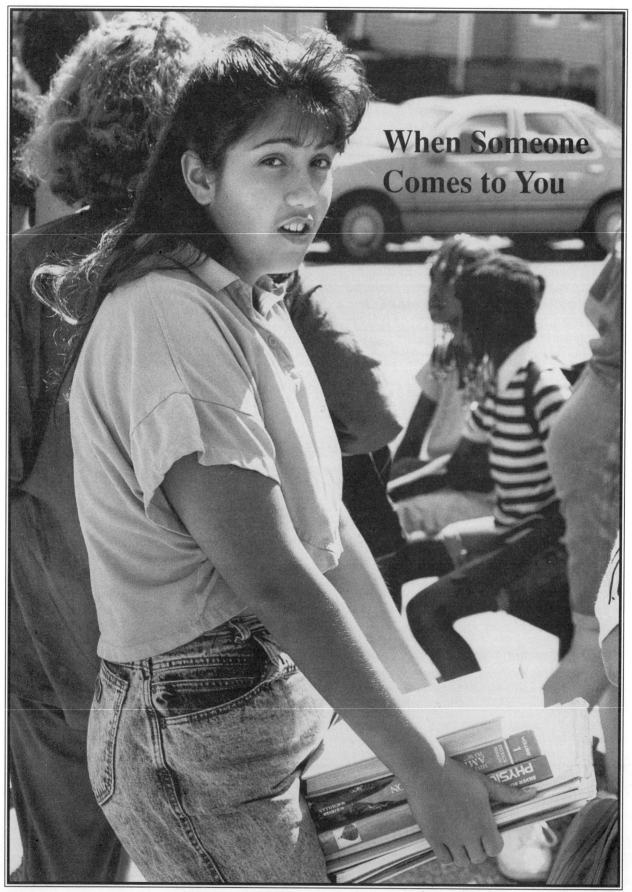

When Someone Comes to You

PHOTO BY JIM WHITMER

When Someone Comes to You: Helping You Minister to Teens

by Anne Van Dillon Roth and Diana L. Hynson

Carpe Diem: Seize the Day

Talk about AIDS in any setting, especially church, makes people uncomfortable because the real issues here are sex, drugs, and death. These are loaded, emotionally gut-wrenching issues for most people in the face of the mere fact of our being human.

Lectures, classes, and workshops lay down foundations of basic information, but the effective moments come very often one-to-one as the young people in our lives carry on their daily agendas. Any conversation in the halls, around the table, over a soda, that touches dating, relationships, parties, drug use, marriage, and children is an opportunity to raise the issue of AIDS.

Of course, the reality is that if you are a trusted adult friend to teens, they may be the ones who bring up the subject first. You need to be ready to deal with the emotional context of that first contact too. Some teens are curious, some are scared, some are struggling with issues of their own sexuality, some may already be sick, some may want to sort out how to talk to their parents.

How you relate to teens is crucial to your potential for success in informing, educating, and caring for them in the face of a deadly threat to their well-being and to their future.

Puberty comes as a storm of sensual awareness, a sometimes terrifying deluge of embarrassing noticings. Teenagers may seem like half-child/half-adult beings who are travelling the unsettling, sometimes agonizing, path to identity. You are aware of their seesaw emotional balance. Buffeted by peers, ads, MTV, delusions of "cool," loud music, the latest styles, the latest fads, a tentative spiritual blooming, and the pervasive fear of not being acceptable, the last thing they need from us is more buffeting and less acceptance. Not every teen rides a perpetual emotional roller coaster, but the culture and identity of teenagers makes these years unique in their path of development.

AIDS impacts every person in our society, and its implications for the youth of this day and their ability to reach maturity are staggering. The best way we can help is through listening and education. The information and exercises in this section will give you at least a beginning handle on how to be a good friend to teens as they confront one of the most terrifying issues in our day. Refer to other segments of this resource for more information on specific issues, like God and AIDS, how to get beyond no, and others.

What, Me Worry?

One of the biggest problems for group leaders dealing with HIV/AIDS topics is being tripped up by their own issues. When we train volunteers to work with people with AIDS, we deliberately push their buttons in a controlled setting during training so that they will have some insight into the questions that will be raised.

✎ Since we can't have each one of you experience the training under ideal conditions, we can at least raise the issues for you to think about here. Ask yourself the following questions. Write down a sentence or two to be sure that you do know how you feel and can put it into words.

1. Have I written my will? If not, why not?
2. Is my Durable Power of Attorney for Health on file with my trusted partner, my doctor, my lawyer?
3. Have I considered my own wishes for my own funeral? Have I communicated those to the person who might be most likely to have to carry them out?
4. Is my insurance adequate to provide for me if I developed a catastrophic illness? Have I considered the possibility in my own life?
5. Have I ever been with someone dear who had a terminal illness? If so, how did I feel about them as soon as I knew they would die?
6. How do I feel about visiting someone with a terminal illness? As the disease changes their looks and their abilities, what does that do to me?
7. Knowing that AIDS is often sexually transmitted, how do I feel about people who have contracted the disease? Am I comfortable sitting next to them?
8. If someone who is or had been a love partner came to me and told me he or she now had AIDS, how would I react to him or her?
9. How do I feel about people who use intravenous drugs? Do I think their addiction is a choice?
10. If my child were to tell me he or she had gotten HIV from a needle, how would I feel?
11. If one of my youth group came to me to ask about condoms, what would I tell him or her?
12. If one of my youth group came to me thinking he or she had contracted the AIDS virus, what would I say?
13. If I overheard young people from my youth group bragging about unsafe sexual activity, what would I say to them?

Life in these decades has made it easy for us to let slide our confrontations with the hard facts. Unless we have had personal contact with terminal illness or had the walls of our immortality/inviolability punctured by an accident or unexpected attack, we can live comfortably within our denial. If we are to be good models and good teachers to our young people who are being asked to deal NOW with these possibilities, we must learn to be brutally honest with ourselves. We are called as Christians to live daily as if we would die gladly tomorrow knowing our home is in heaven.

Models of God and Christian Responsibility

Though of paramount importance, it is not enough to think through only how we feel about terminal illness, at-risk behavior, and the social implications of being ill. If we are to be ministers to youth, in addition to mentors or trusted friends, we must help them think theologically about who they are, whose they are, and what they do.

The biblical characterizations of God are numerous, and we will not examine all of them, but the ones that follow will help you sort out how to speak to teens about who God is and how God relates to us. Use a study Bible and a commentary to help you understand these references.

✎ Read through these Scripture passages and then ask yourself:

✤ Is this a way that I understand and can relate to God? What are the personal "pictures" or images of God? How can I see myself in each relationship with God that the image suggests?
✤ Can I interpret this to a teenager? What would I say?
✤ What personal example can I recall or create that will help this image of God be "real" for a teen?

God Provides and Loves: God has provided for us richly and loves us so much that God cannot forsake us, no matter what the cost to God. (**Isaiah 49:8-23, John 3:16-21, 1 John 4:7-21**)

God Guards and Protects: God wants us to be safe from all sin and all evils and protects us. (**Psalms 91 and 121; Isaiah 40:10-11, 27-31; John 17:6-19**)

God Heals and Cares: God is able to heal all diseases (sometimes through death) and cares for and about us. (**Psalm 23, 2 Corinthians 1:3-4, Matthew 12:9-21, John 11:17-44**)

God Confronts and Holds Us Accountable: Though God loves us faithfully, we cannot do just anything against the will of God. God knows the sin we do and expects us to repent and change. (**2 Samuel 11-12, Luke 13:22-35, John 8:1-11, Hebrews 12:1-13**)

God Forgives and Offers Hope: Though we are judged for what we do, God always provides the hope for repentance and salvation. (**Psalm 103, Isaiah 40:1-11, Acts 2:14-39, Galatians 6:1-10**)

God Promises Life and Eternal Life: God has acted through the ages and through Jesus Christ to provide all that we need for life and forever. (**John 6:35-40, John 10:22-30, Revelation 22:1-7**)

One danger in speaking and analyzing from a theological perspective is losing our balance. God is neither the God who only judges harshly and punishes swiftly, nor the God who blindly loves, forgives, and condones. Grace is a wonderful gift of God, but it is not cheap. You have the Christian responsibility to hold up this creative tension for teenagers and to help explain and explore with them what it means in terms of their own values, behaviors, and beliefs.

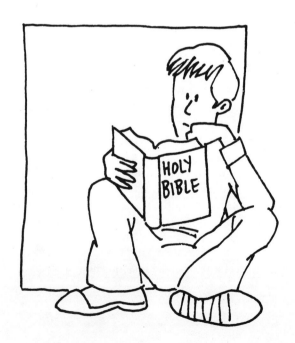

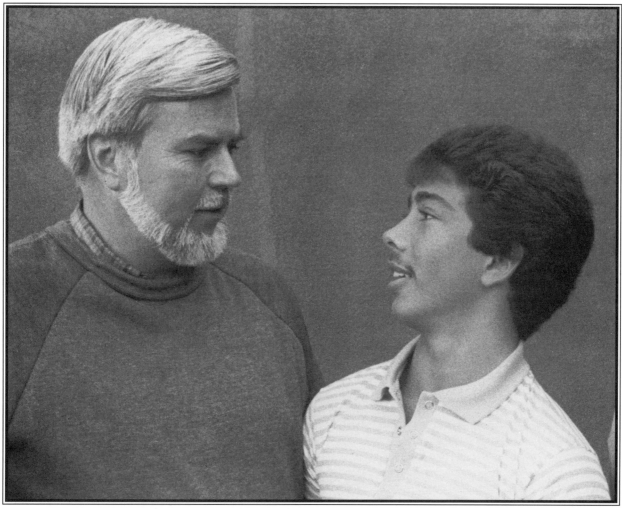

PHOTO BY MIMI FORSYTH

Family Systems

You may be called upon to relate to the families of your teens in a variety of ways. Some obvious possibilities include keeping them informed of any formal or intentional educational plans (such as using this resource); interceding for/with a teen who needs to inform his or her parents about the results of risky behavior and can't or won't talk to them alone; or inviting them to family/teen conversations about sex, drugs, and AIDS.

You may also be asked by a teen to talk about his or her sexuality or sexual orientation. That teen may have no intention of discussing the same subject at home, and you have a delicate task in determining how to proceed. It is not within the scope of this resource to deal with issues of "coming out" or sexuality, except as it relates to AIDS, and we can only suggest that you consult a sympathetic professional for guidance.

Family systems in the United States are vastly different than they were a generation or so ago. The many changes in the family unit foster unique circumstances in understanding and dealing with families, especially if they are configured differently than our own.

✎ As you think through how to relate to the various family units of your teens, ask yourself these questions.

✤ How well do I know the parents or guardians?
✤ Who is the head of the household?
✤ What do I know about the recent history of this family that would help me understand them better?
✤ Am I familiar with the culture and language of this family? If not, how could I become better acquainted?
✤ What do I know about the values of this family? If I am unfamiliar with them, how could I become better acquainted?
✤ What differences and similarities might I expect between my age, gender, generation, educational level, and position and that of the family?
✤ How can I make good use of the strengths and cope maturely with the challenges?
✤ How can I cultivate and maintain an atmosphere of mutual respect and trust?

Just Like Me . . .

The most effective AIDS educators we have used in the local high school education programs have been peers of the students, either students themselves or young adults who have gone through the advanced training. The key person seems to be a personable young man I'll call Bill. He is now in his early 20's, looks younger, and his HIV has advanced to the ARC stage. His symptoms are not readily visible, but they have taken sufficient toll that his description of his journey through HIV is believable. He is considered "cute" by the high school girls and therefore pulls their sympathy readily.

Bringing the reality of HIV "home" to young people seems to be the difficulty. Those of us who are adults and authority figures to them are all too easily discounted. Usually the word of peers is taken seriously and sometimes the shock of their experience and circumstances has value. Consider the following true story to see how sharing a personal experience can reach a young person. Consider also calling a local AIDS hotline or service for the name of willing teen speakers who can relate to your youth.

Never Doing Anything

At an educational fair on a college campus a young black woman approached the table where I sat.

"AIDS! I don't need to know nothing about AIDS."

"Why not?" I asked immediately.

"'Cause I'm never doing anything to get it," was her flippant reply as she deliberately walked away from me.

"What a lonely life," I said, and it stopped her in her tracks.

As a black woman, she is 25-33% more likely to encounter HIV in her life than a white woman of her age group. Any man she hopes to marry, any children she hopes to have are in a high risk category simply by virtue of the social structure in this country.

Her greatest danger: "I don't need to know . . ."

In this case a fast comeback at least made her stop and think. If she had been more willing to talk and less fearful, it would have been interesting to get her to list out loud the behaviors she knew were safe and to help her to understand that "never doing anything" in her situation could include never having a child, never finding a husband. It's not easy to know when and what has to be risked or how to lessen the risk.

You need to know. They need to know. Anyone who has made love with another person or shared a hypodermic needle in the last ten years in this country is potentially at risk for HIV. We all need to know what the risks are and are not.

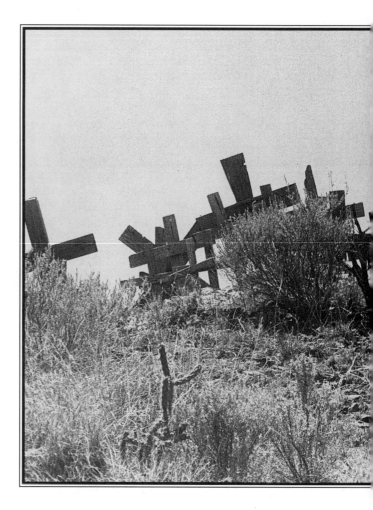

Tough Love, Tough Truth

We are seeing a curious phenomenon in the world of HIV as it affects young people. In two years (1989-91) there has been a 77% increase in the number of cases of AIDS among people ages 17-22. Why? Where were these people when Health class was in session? Don't they know about AIDS?

Yes. Sort of. It appears that the denial of the adults who have done the telling and the teaching has had a heavy impact on the teen's understanding of what HIV does. We are seeing newly diagnosed clients with HIV who were never told the hard news: AIDS can kill you. AIDS is fatal. There's no cure.

"Because the pandemic is not under control anywhere, physicians from everywhere urge the need to do the only thing guaranteed to stop transmission—get people to change their sexual and drug-injecting behavior." (*Journal of the American Medical Association*, Sept. 9, 1992; Vol. 268: pages 1237-1246.)

As the number of full-blown AIDS cases in the United States reaches the quarter-million mark, the numbers begin to stagger. A recent television report on AIDS and Teens (Channel 2 San Francisco, 10 P.M. Sept. 17,

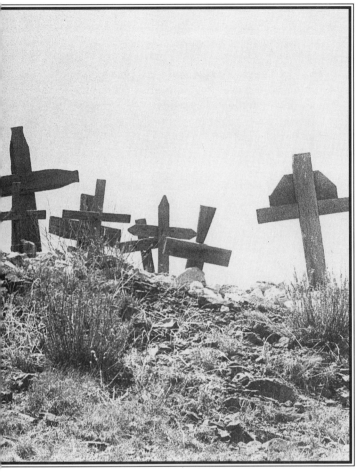

PHOTO BY MIMI FORSYTH

AIDS Ain't Pretty

➤ HIV strips its victims not only of their protective immunity to the ravages of diseases, but also of dignity, independence, appetite, friends, family, and even their own minds. Clusters of parasites and fungi invade their bodies and rob them of the ability to eat or gain nourishment from what they eat. As they starve slowly to death, their very muscles are consumed. That is why the Africans call this the "Skinny Disease." It causes intense suffering.

➤ The cancer associated with HIV, Kaposi's Sarcoma (KS) creates dark swellings in the blood vessels and eventually in the major organs. It kills by interfering with the body's functions, and it is very painful.

➤ Pneumocystic Carinii Pneumonia (PCP) drowns its victims in lung fluid. It is caused by a protozoan that lives in most healthy human bodies and is normally kept under control by the immune system. Not being able to breathe hurts. A lot.

➤ Other diseases drain HIV positive bodies with diarrhea and blister their brains with lesions. When HIV moves into brain tissue, the result is a dementia very like that of Alzheimer's Disease. Not being able to control yourself feels terrible.

1992) gave statistics that African American teens are eleven times more likely to be diagnosed with AIDS than white teens and Hispanic teens three times more likely. When an African American girl was asked what it would take to change the pattern, she answered, "early comprehensive AIDS education with role models."

A well-known AIDS counsellor in our area got a phone call one evening from a 21-year-old man. He'd had sex once in his life, and now he is HIV positive.

➤ HIV ruins your love life.
➤ HIV ruins your looks.
➤ HIV ruins any hope you may have of having healthy children.
➤ HIV ruins your future.

The plight of that 21-year-old man will strike home best if someone in that situation is the one that expresses it to the teens, because most youth have a powerful (and erroneous) concept of their own immortality and invulnerability, which directly feeds the "It can't happen to me" mind set. If the personal stories do not claim attention, perhaps some of the gory medical details will. Consider those that follow.

➤ HIV is a "smart" virus. Once it enters your blood stream, it mutates to suit your system. You may think it doesn't matter once you're infected if you continue a sexual relationship with a partner who is already infected, but it does. The virus mutates to suit your partner's body too. And *every time* you share the virus, you're getting another version. Reinfection speeds death, causes endless complications, and worsens any chance you might have to survive. Lovemaking becomes death-making.

No one should have to die this way—and no one has to with a little common sense! Our greatest danger is in our ability to lie to ourselves.

Risk-taking around AIDS is

NOT smart

NOT macho

NOT wise.

If your teens have to prove themselves by doing scary things, encourage them to take up public speaking or collect snakes.

Building Support to "Just Say No"

No one in the history of the world has succeeded in legislating morality for humans, including the church, although at its best our faith offers an exemplary example of how to live, believe, and behave in ways that honor God, each other, and ourselves.

That notwithstanding, many young people demonstrate some innate sense of their own immortality, and that sense erodes their caution or common sense. Some teens just do not realize that painful, unalterable results can come from risky behavior. Many fail to either understand or take seriously the consequences of what they do.

Some teens have such weak images of their self-worth or such poor support systems at home, school, or even church, that they are ill-equipped to resist the negative pressure from peers or elsewhere to engage in at-risk activities. For these, and many other teens, telling them "don't" doesn't work.

What can you do to help shore up those support systems so that teens can recognize and resist temptation? One avenue, as mentioned earlier, is to do all in your power to get teens' attention and trust so that you can provide information. Ignorance is a powerful weapon against good physical, emotional, and spiritual health. Then what?

Search Institute (Minneapolis, MN) in its December 1990 and April 1991 issues of *Source* (a quarterly information resource on issues facing children, adolescents, and families) has identified internal and external assets that teens need from others for support until they mature enough to cultivate these assets for themselves. As an adult friend to youth, you are in a good position to help provide these supports.

External Assets—Support: family support, parents as social resources, parent communication, parental involvement in schooling, other adult communication, other adult resources, a positive school climate.

External Assets—Control: parental standards, discipline, monitoring; time at home; positive peer influence.

External Assets—Structured Use of Time: involved in music, school extracurricular activities, community organizations, church, or synagogue.

Internal Assets—Educational Commitment: school performance, achievement motivation, serious about homework, aspiration to education.

Internal Assets—Positive Values: values related to sexual restraint and helping people, concern about world hunger and poverty, care about others' feelings.

Internal Assets—Social Competence: self-esteem; assertiveness, decision-making, friend-making, and planning skills; a positive view of personal future.

Almost all of these factors can be influenced positively if the adults surrounding youth are willing and find it important enough to do so. Teens with these internal and external supports are much more likely to listen, consider consequences, and resist negative peer pressure that puts them at risk.

On the practical level, you need to recognize and have a response to all the excuses and mythical thinking that teens buy into. What others can you add to this sampling and what would you say?
➤ But he or she said I was the first.
➤ I'm safe.
➤ It can't happen to me.
➤ My partner wouldn't do that to me.
➤ Once won't hurt.
➤ I don't need to use a condom; besides, it takes away the pleasure or takes too long, or I forget, or . . .
➤ He or she didn't look sick.
➤ I've known him or her for years; everything's cool.
➤ I'm the last living virgin at my school!

Numerous other practical helps are included in other sections of this resource. See especially "Saying No to Sex," page 9; "AIDS and Drugs," pages 16-17; "Dealing With Denial," pages 24-26; the video, *Spread the Word*; and *What You Can Do to Avoid AIDS* by Magic Johnson.

The HIV Loss Exercise

This exercise is an elaboration of a training exercise used by the nurses and that we have built into one of the most effective experiences of our considerable training. When we do this exercise at the AIDS Project of Contra Costa with 45 to 80 trainees who are preparing to be "buddies" to people with HIV disease, there has been a consistent deeply emotional response from many of the participants. For some, it is their first encounter with "loss of control" in their own existence and shatters the easy denial that most of us live with. It has been helpful to have trained facilitators immediately available to these people to help them unpack the experience. Adapt this exercise to your group size and available space.

✎ You will need:
Packages of self-sticking labels
Marker pens for everyone
Boxes of kleenex ·

✎ Have a small number of participants be the "HIV Virus." They will wait while the others do the following activities:

✎ Give each participant twelve to sixteen labels. Have them write several labels for each of the following categories: special people in their lives, favorite possessions, favorite activities, hoped-for dreams and goals.

✎ Have them stick the labels all over their chest and arms, then pair off. Each partner should have a few minutes to look at the other's list of things; each partner should have a few minutes to describe what the meaning is for them of their various labels.

✎ The leader then explains that HIV coming into someone's life forces them to lose important parts of themselves. Ask each person voluntarily to take off one label, "give it up." Give them a minute to think about that.

✎ As HIV moves in to begin to destroy the immune system, more things are lost: Ask each person to remove one more label.

✎ At this point release the assigned "HIV people" to wander among the participants removing labels randomly. Give them time to circle the group. Expect emotional reactions from some people.

✎ Have the "HIV people" gather in one corner of the room or space. Then start the discussion by asking participants to respond to the experience:
✦ What was taken? How did that feel? How did they feel about the one who did the taking? How did they feel about what happened to their partner?

✎ When there are no further comments, ask the "HIV people" to describe how they felt taking the labels.
✦ Did they look people in the eye? Did they crumple up the labels or treat them gently?

✎ Lead the discussion to the direct effect on people's lives of a slowly-debilitating disease like HIV/AIDS that runs to an inevitable end. This exercise is designed to awaken their awareness of what people with HIV are experiencing in their lives—the uncontrollable, inexorable loss that leads to ultimate loss of life.

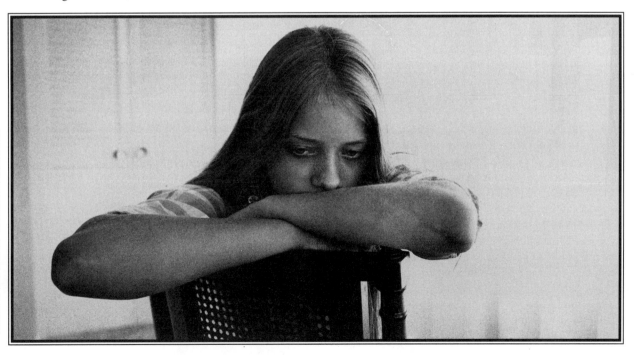

PHOTO BY JEAN-CLAUDE LEJEUNE

Bedside Manners: When the End Is Near

AIDS is no respecter of age nor station. As an adult worker and friend with youth, you may be called upon to be at the bedside of a teen or teen's family member as he or she faces death. Facing death is no easy task, either at the beginning when a diagnosis of HIV is confirmed, or at the end when what is probably a premature death is inevitable. You will be asked, or will feel the need, to help others make some meaning out of these eternal issues of life and death. Have you faced any of the issues around your own mortality? Do you have an understanding of and a relationship with Christ that helps you release the fear of death and trust that your life now and life after life are in God's hands?

These are heavy questions, but you must try to address them at least for yourself. Certainly, these are questions for which our answers will be incomplete, but preparing yourself is crucial for being a helpful Christian friend to another person.

The personal story that follows may give you insight to that time and place we all pray will never come and we fear will not come. We do not have to have formal training to be a loving presence to one who is seriously ill or dying, but we do have to have some sensitivity for when to "do something" and when to be quiet.

Those of us who work among the people with AIDS learn quickly, Christian or not, to leave behind any punitive dogmas of religion. Our task is to succor, not to judge. We are in the picture of their lives as a silent Samaritan who never questioned the belief system of the man he helped. He simply listened, cared, and paid the bill.

We also pay the bill with the gifts of acceptance, listening, and the stifling of our own agendas. We bear the nail prints of our own griefs. We put ourselves through heavy-duty training, trying to learn as much as we can about the disease and the implications, and then we work one-on-one with people in need.

We sit in theaters or restaurants with our buddies, a friend available for an outing that is good for the soul. We sit on park benches and in living rooms, sharing moments and feelings. We sit in waiting rooms and hospitals, available for errands or hugs. We sit, eventually, at bedsides to help change a T-shirt soaked with night sweats, to be a strong arm for someone who needs to go once again to the bathroom, to dance a dance of support while a bed is changed. We sometimes sleep in their rooms when they are afraid to be alone, afraid of the dark, afraid of the darkness to come.

And we witness. We witness their increasing debility, their fear, their weaknesses, their ravaged feelings, their strength and courage and wondrous love as they prepare to leave this world. We are careful to understand their need for "religious talk," and when to leave that alone. If we are wise, we witness to them with our presence, our caring, and if they are willing, with our spoken prayers. In return, we reap the priceless gift of sharing in their launch into the next life, which for many is a great unknown.

I spent Thursday after Thursday with my friend, one of a whole calendar of volunteers who spent regular time with this man who did not want to be alone—ever. I watched a beautiful 6-foot-tall man go from 165 pounds down to 92, from being the leading light of a group of persons with AIDS to being too weak to speak. He was concerned: he said he didn't know how to die. He wasn't sure he could state this as meticulously as he had staged so many parties and events for others.

I spent one night in his room when his regular night respite care person was away, and we were companionable in the darkness. He couldn't die. He couldn't let go. As the process dragged on, one concerned friend who knew well of his habit of keeping a day book said the problem was that no one had put on his calendar: Today would be a good day to die. We laughed, and inside we held our breath. Could he do it? Could he let go?

For someone who said he didn't know how, he did an incredible job. The evening he died, he was holding his mother's hand and the music on the TV in the background was "Amazing Grace." On the day he was buried, we threw him the party he'd wanted us to have.

One year ago this week he died, and I miss him still; jokes I can't share, flowers he'd love to plant, and stories to tell. And he knew when he nursed his own partner who died of AIDS that his day would come.

What about you? If you are feeling too overwhelmed or inadequate for the task of being in ministry to teens, whether they are ill from the complications of HIV/AIDS or are simply curious, remember this:

➤ Kindness is rarely misplaced. How would you want to be treated in a similar circumstance?

➤ Love and trust are more important than reproof, but be sensitive to those occasions when confrontation is the most loving thing to do.

➤ Prayer is always appropriate. If praying out loud is not a good idea in a given situation, God hears your silent prayers too.

➤ You are not alone; God is always present to guide you. Ask for help.

Anne Van Dillen Roth has worked in a variety of roles with AIDS Project of Contra Costa in Walnut Creek, CA, for over three years. She was ordained in the Southern New Jersey Conference of The United Methodist Church in 1977 and 1979 and served ten years as a pastor before moving to California with her husband. She is currently doing part-time parish administration for another church as well as writing.

Diana L. Hynson is an editor with the Department of Youth Publications at The United Methodist Publishing House in Nashville, TN. Diana has edited and contributed to several youth publications.

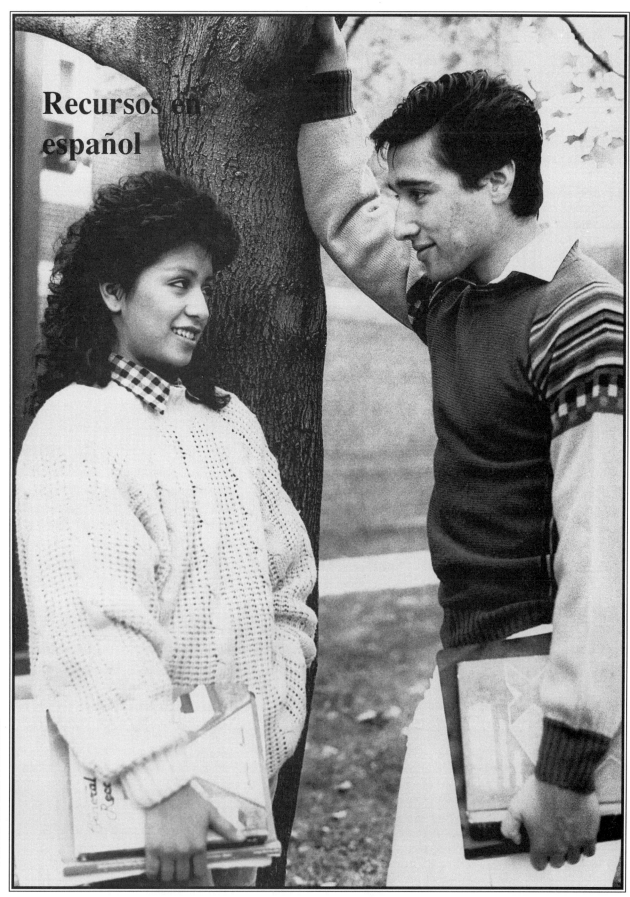

Recursos en español

PHOTO BY JIM WHITMER

¿Qué tiene que ver la iglesia con el SIDA?

por Carmen M. Gaud

¿De qué trata este recurso?

El recurso que tiene en sus manos ha sido escrito con el propósito de proveer a los líderes y maestros de la juventud en nuestras iglesias una guía de estudio sobre el SIDA. Si vivimos según los principios de vida que el Evangelio establece, las personas cristianas confiamos que enfermedades como el SIDA no nos toquen. Desgraciadamente no hay garantías absolutas de que no nos toquen. Lo que comenzó en algunos lugares como una enfermedad de un grupo específico, los homosexuales, se ha convertido en una de las crisis de salud más serias con las que se está enfrentando el mundo en estos momentos.

El SIDA no es una enfermedad de homosexuales. Las personas con adicción a drogas, los hemofílicos, y los matrimonios se han ido añadiendo a la lista de personas que padecen de HIV/SIDA. El riesgo de contaminación se ha ido multiplicando con el tiempo a causa de las características de la enfermedad. Conocer estas características y saber qué se puede hacer para prevenir el problema puede hacer la diferencia entre la vida y la muerte.

¿Por qué se debe tratar este tema?

Mi primer encuentro con el SIDA ocurrió hace algunos años. Conocí a una hermana en la fe, muy activa en su congregación, mano derecha de la pastora de la iglesia. Tanto ella como su marido habían tenido una experiencia muy profunda de fe. El marido de esta hermana había usado drogas pero, en el momento que lo conocí, su vida había sido renovada en Cristo. Comenzó a tener lo que creyó que era un simple catarro. Al pasar el tiempo sin que se curara, el médico quiso hacer más pruebas. Descubrieron que su condición era SIDA.

Después que su marido murió, la esposa se casó nuevamente y tuvo una niña de este matrimonio. Un tiempo después, su segundo marido desarrolló el SIDA, al igual que su niña. Este segundo marido murió, después la niña y, finalmente, esta hermana cristiana. Al morir esta hermana, dejó varios hijos e hijas de diferentes edades, fruto de su matrimonio anterior. ¿Cómo llamarse persona cristiana y no tener misericordia de los que sufren?

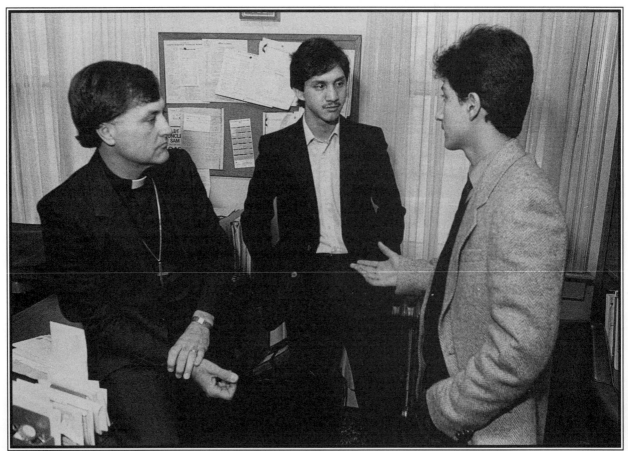

PHOTO BY SID DORRIS

¿Cuán grave es el problema?

Después de esa experiencia han sucedido muchas otras cosas en el mundo. En 1991 la televisión nos dejó ver los rostros de miles de bebés rumanos con SIDA a consecuencia de las prácticas médicas en Rumania. Debido a la limitación de equipo médico, los hospitales rumanos estaban usando agujas hipodérmicas sin desinfectarlas en forma apropiada. Como consecuencia, miles de bebés fueron infectados.

En 1992 se dió a conocer en Francia la práctica irresponsable de médicos que, aún sabiendo que la sangre estaba infectada con el virus HIV, permitieron su uso en tranfusiones de sangre. Cientos de personas con hemofilia recibieron las transfusiones, algunos de los cuales ya habían muerto al momento del juicio. La situación en Francia ha sido semejante a la de muchos otros pacientes, infectados por transfusiones de sangre.

¿Qué puede hacer la iglesia?

A consecuencia de mi primera experiencia con el SIDA, y del conocimiento de las otras, creó que cada congregación debe estar preparada para enfrentarse a esta enfermedad. Cada congregación debe preparar a su membresía con información que le ayude a prevenir la enfermedad; debe estar lista para ministrar a los pacientes de SIDA, sea que lleguen a sus puertas o que estén dentro de las mismas; y debe asegurarse que todas las edades reciban información. No debemos cerrar los ojos a la situación y encontrarnos con que somos culpables de participar en la crisis.

¿Cómo se debe usar el recurso?

Creo que el recurso se hace más útil si:

➤ Los líderes responsables de la educación de la juventud tienen oportunidad de estudiar este recurso en su totalidad.

➤ Los líderes deciden cuáles de los programas que se incluyen, tanto en inglés como en castellano, son más útiles para la juventud de su congregación.

➤ Los líderes discuten sus planes con el pastor o pastora de la iglesia, con otros miembros de la Junta Administrativa, y con los padres de los jóvenes a quienes quiere incluir en el estudio.

¿Por qué las personas adultas?

El tema y la forma tan abierta en que se discuten ciertos asuntos hace necesario el apoyo de las personas adultas. Los padres y las madres de sus alumnos y alumnas deben comprender el propósito de estos programas. Deben, además, recibir información que les ayude personalmente. Hay muchos mitos y falsa información sobre el SIDA que debe ser aclarado. Este recurso trata de incluir información reciente sobre el SIDA y de orientar a las personas adultas tanto como a la juventud. Además da información que es útil para los grupos y congregaciones que desean ministrar a personas afectadas por la enfermedad.

Si es posible, algunos padres pueden trabajar junto con el maestro o la maestra, como ayudantes en las sesiones. Vea las recomendaciones para la enseñanza que cada sesión incluye. Adapte cuanto sea necesario para que sus jóvenes aprovechen al máximo la experiencia educativa que se le está proponiendo a su grupo. Asegúrese de que sus jóvenes reciban la mejor calidad de enseñanza posible. Usted y su congregación pueden hacer un gran impacto entre la juventud y en su comunidad.

¿Qué más se debe saber?

Como ya se habrá dado cuenta, este recurso es en inglés y en castellano. Muchas de las iglesias en que se usará el recurso tienen grupos bilingues de jóvenes. Aún los maestros y maestras pueden tener dificultad en el manejo del castellano. En otras congregaciones, sin embargo, el idioma principal será el castellano.

Nos interesa que la información llegue a la juventud en el lenguaje y la forma que sea más efectiva. Usted, como líder, puede ayudar a adaptar cada sesión para que se aplique a su grupo. Las sesiones en castellano han sido escritas por personas hispanas que conocen el problema y que están involucradas en la solución del mismo. Su enfoque va dirigido a la población hispana en Estados Unidos y Puerto Rico. La parte en inglés también incluye temas que pueden ser muy necesarios para nuestros jóvenes. Léalos y úselos como crea conveniente.

¿Cómo usar este recurso?

Este recurso fue aprobado como material en inglés solamente. Debido a la urgencia que existe de educar a la juventud sobre el tema del SIDA, se tomó la decisión de añadir un número de páginas adicionales que sirvieran a las comunidades hispanas en los Estados Unidos y Puerto Rico. Se diseñaron los programas en castellano con la intención de abordar el tema desde una perspectiva pastoral hispana. Por otra parte, esperamos que las congregaciones bilingues y las que deseen usar los artículos y recursos en inglés aprovechen todo el material.

Hay artículos e historias en inglés que pueden ser usadas por congregaciones cuyo idioma principal es el castellano. El maestro o maestra puede traducir alguna de las historias y escoger las actividades educativas más apropiadas para su grupo. Los programas de este libro no requieren que los alumnos y alumnas tengan copias del libro. En algunos casos encontrará que se da permiso para la reproducción del material. Lo más importante es que la información llegue a nuestra juventud.

El material puede ser usado en diferentes formas y lugares. Puede ser parte del programa de un grupo de estudio. Puede usarse como parte de un retiro de jóvenes o de las reuniones de la sociedad de jóvenes. Las secciones *Programs* y *More Program Ideas*, así como los titulados *Programas* en castellano están diseñados para un formato tradicional de estudio.

Tanto en inglés como en castellano, los artículos ("Teaching Articles"), los guías para el líder ("Leader's Guides") y la sección final pueden ayudarle si desea ampliar el tema. Le provee datos sobre otros recursos impresos y humanos con los que puede contar. Tanto en los Estados Unidos como en Puerto Rico usted puede solicitar la participación de alguna de estas agencias para ofrecer mayor información a su congregación o a su grupo de jóvenes.

Lo que puede resultarle más difícil de adaptar puede ser la sección en inglés dedicada a los líderes: "Leader's Guides". Las películas y el libro a los que se refieren las guías no están disponibles en castellano. Puede ser necesario que usted diseñe otra forma de presentar el material que se discute en estos recursos.

El tema del SIDA es complicado y controversial. Tratar en forma superficial los asuntos no va a ayudar a nuestra juventud. El reto ante usted es grande. Oramos para que en su congregación este recurso sea recibido como medio de reflexionar acerca de una situación crítica. Pedimos a Dios que las advertencias que se presentan a nuestra juventud los ayuden a madurar en sus decisiones y a escoger unos estilos de vida que sean productivos y sanos, en armonía con la vida abundante que nuestro Dios desea para sus hijos e hijas.

SU IGLESIA PUEDE HACER LA DIFERENCIA ENTRE LA VIDA Y LA MUERTE!

Carmen M. Gaud es ministro ordenada de la Iglesia Metodista de Puerto Rico. Ha trabajado desde 1986 como editora de Recursos de Currículum en español de la Casa Metodista Unida de Publicaciones.

Programa:
¿Qué sabe nuestra juventud sobre el HIV/SIDA?

por Eliecel Rodríguez

Introducción

Este programa tiene como propósito general educar a nuestra juventud sobre el HIV/SIDA. Desde el 1981 se comenzó a hablar mucho sobre el SIDA. Muchas personas comenzaron a manifestar los síntomas característicos de la enfermedad del SIDA. El sistema inmunológico de las personas con síntomas estaba casi destruido.

El SIDA (el resultado de la infección por el virus HIV) cada día ataca a mayor número de personas, y amenaza con destruir a nuestra juventud. Aunque los tratamientos médicos han mejorado en los últimos años, los científicos opinan que aún faltan muchos años más para una cura. Si queremos evitar que la epidemia del HIV/SIDA continue, tendremos que recurrir á la mejor solución que existe hasta el momento, la educación.

El programa tratará de enseñar a la juventud cómo protegerse del contagio con SIDA. El programa está basado en los siguientes conceptos:

➤ El HIV/SIDA es una enfermedad mortal contra la cual no se ha descubierto ninguna cura.
➤ Tanto la juventud como las personas adultas pueden evitar el contagio con HIV/SIDA.
➤ Hay ciertas actividades y conductas que representan mayor riesgo de contraer el virus HIV y finalmente el SIDA.
➤ El conocer y tomar ciertas precauciones pueden ayudar a la juventud a evitar el contraer la enfermedad.

Preparación para la sesión

✎ Tenga a mano una cartulina para la clase, y papeles en blanco tamaño carta para cada alumno. Consiga marcadores y lápices para escribir.

✎ Lea el programa completo antes de comenzar. Familiarícese con los propósitos y conceptos principales.

✎ Solicite de antemano copias de folletos y otros materiales impresos sobre HIV/SIDA y téngalos disponibles para repartir durante la reunión.

✎ Si la mayoría de los jóvenes en su grupo son menores de 15 años, puede desarrollar la sesión como una búsqueda de datos. Coloque la información en tarjetas o use los impresos que haya recibido. Distribuya los datos en el salón. Escriba las oraciones del Ejercicio 1 en la pizarra o en una cartulina. Cada alumno(a) debe buscar en el salón los datos e ir respondiendo a las oraciones. Cuando todos hayan terminado, reúnalos y déles la oportunidad de compartir lo que descubrieron.

✎ Si la mayor parte de su grupo está formado por mayores de 15 años puede variar la búsqueda de datos. Asigne temas por grupos pequeños y permítales buscar los datos en las tarjetas o impresos. Cada grupo presentará su informe al grupo total. Haga las preguntas del Ejercicio 1 al terminar los informes.

✎ Si usa el método de búsqueda de datos en su grupo, haga el Ejercicio 2 al principio del programa para ayudar a los jóvenes a comprender la seriedad de la epidemia. Tanto al principio como al final del programa es importante recalcar la seriedad de la epidemia y la importancia de la prevención.

✎ Reserve algún tiempo al final del programa para evaluar el aprendizaje logrado por el grupo.

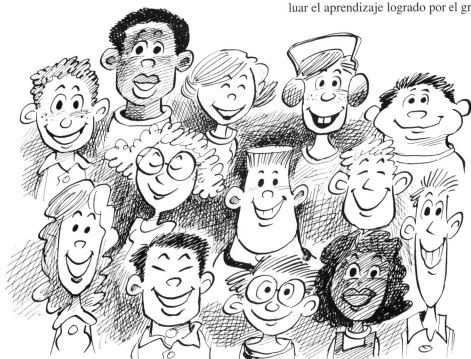

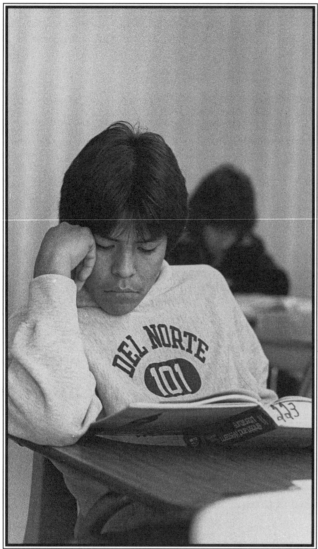

PHOTO BY MIMI FORSYTH

Tome en cuenta la audiencia

Cuando se le habla a la juventud en forma autoritaria, los jóvenes se resisten a escuchar. Sea cordial siempre y nunca juzgue a su audiencia en forma negativa. Su función como instructor(a) es muy importante.

Al hablar del HIV/SIDA con un grupo juvenil usted tiene que hablar sobre el sexo, las drogas, y la muerte. Estos temas pueden ser muy difíciles de tratar, pero se tienen que enfrentar si se quiere ayudar a la juventud.

Es muy común en la juventud el creerse invencible y que nada malo le puede pasar a uno. En esta época llena de riesgos, cualquier error puede ser devastador para la vida de una persona joven.

El objetivo de este programa es educar y dar opciones a nuestra juventud hispana para evitar que contraigan el HIV/SIDA. Como instructor(a) usted debe separar sus prejuicios e ideas personales de los datos concretos sobre el problema. Lo importante es que la enseñanza/aprendizaje pueda llevarse a cabo.

Ejercicio 1

✎ Reparta a sus alumnos y alumnas un papel y un lápiz para este ejercicio. Haga un ejercicio de cierto y falso. Pida a los alumnos(as) que doblen el papel en dos partes. Deben contestar el ejercicio usando el doblez superior. Al final del programa de hoy, contestarán el ejercicio nuevamente, usando el doblez interior. Bríndeles la oportunidad de corregir los datos que conocen sobre el SIDA.

1) El HIV no tiene nada que ver con la enfermedad de SIDA. (Falso)
2) El SIDA se contagia si uno toca a una persona infectada. (Falso)
3) Las relaciones sexuales con una persona enferma con HIV/SIDA pueden contagiar a su compañero o compañera. (Cierto)
4) Algunos bebés se contagian porque sus mamás están enfermas con HIV/SIDA. (Cierto)
5) La mejor manera de evitar el contagio con HIV/SIDA es no tener relaciones sexuales. (Cierto)
6) Es conveniente conocer quienes han sido los compañeros(as) sexuales de personas con las cuales hay planes de tener contacto sexual. (Cierto)
7) Las personas con adicción a drogas no tienen riesgo de contraer HIV/SIDA. (Falso)
8) Un sólo contacto sexual o el compartir la misma aguja una vez no ofrece ningun riesgo. (Falso)
9) Sólo los homosexuales tienen HIV/SIDA. (Falso)
10) Hay recursos y agencias en distintos lugares que pueden ayudar a quienes sospechan que tienen HIV/SIDA. (Cierto)

Le recomendamos que discuta los datos sobre HIV/SIDA en forma oral con el grupo. Para reforzar la enseñanza, puede hacer uso de letreros que prepare previamente con los datos principales o pidiendo algunos de los recursos impresos en castellano que se mencionan en la sección *Solamente los hechos*.

¿Qué es el HIV?

El HIV, el virus de inmunodeficiencia humana, es el virus que causa el SIDA. El virus pasa de una persona a otra por contacto sexual o por transmisión sanguínea. El virus causa varias síntomas en el cuerpo. El resultado de esta infección se conoce como el SIDA.

¿Qué es el SIDA?

El SIDA es el resultado de la infección por el HIV. La infección es causada por un virus (HIV). Cuando una persona desarrolla el SIDA, su sistema inmunológico está afectado y, por lo tanto, no puede combatir otras infecciones. Actualmente estas infecciones son fatales.

Transmisión y prevención

Hay casos documentados de transmisión por los siguientes fluídos corporales.

➤ Sangre
➤ Semen
➤ Secreción vaginal
➤ Leche materna (Pocos casos notificados)

¿Cómo se transmite el HIV?

➤ A través del contacto sexual con una persona infectada.
➤ Al compartir agujas con una persona infectada.
➤ Durante el embarazo, parto o lactancia materna, la madre puede infectar a su hijo o hija.

¿Quién contrae HIV/SIDA?

Personas que están en contacto con la sangre, el semen, o las secreciones vaginales de una persona infectada.

¿Qué puedo hacer para evitar el contraer HIV/SIDA?

➤ No tener relaciones sexuales de ningun tipo (oral, vaginal, anal).
➤ Tener relaciones sexuales solamente con una persona no infectada, monógamas (que no tienen ninguna otra pareja), y que no hayan compartido agujas hipodérmicas con nadie.
➤ Evitar el uso de drogas, especialmente aquellas que requieren uso de agujas hipodérmicas.
➤ Usar condones de látex con espermicida (nonoxynol-9) si va a tener algún contacto sexual.

Como cristianos creemos que la sexualidad es un don de Dios. Como don, debe ser usado en forma saludable, responsable y amorosa. El consejo que debemos dar a la juventud es que es mejor abstenerse de relaciones sexuales antes del matrimonio.

Si hay jóvenes en el grupo que se sospecha mantienen relaciones sexuales, aconseje al menos la protección mediante el uso de condones de látex. Estos disminuyen el riesgo de la infección por HIV. Para más protección deben comprar condones con nonoxynol-9. Nonoxynol-9 es un espermicida que en algunas investigaciones se ha comprobado que disminuye el riesgo de contraer el HIV/SIDA. Recuérdeles que el uso de condones no ofrece un 100% de garantía. Lo más seguro para evitar la infección es no tener relaciones sexuales.

Es muy conveniente conocer las actividades y relaciones sexuales del compañero o compañera, especialmente si hay planes de casamiento. El HIV/SIDA no da señales de su presencia de inmediato. Las actividades sexuales previas pueden no tener consecuencias hasta después de varios años. El conocer los riesgos antes del casamiento puede evitar las sorpresas después.

¿Puedo contraer el HIV/SIDA besando en la boca?

Los besos prolongados pueden dañar la boca y los labios. Esto puede causar que el HIV pase de una persona infectada a otra. Esto sucede al entrar el virus al flujo sanguíneo a través de llagas o cortaduras en la boca y los labios. Sin embargo, no hay casos documentados de transmisión del HIV por medio de un beso en la boca.

Ejercicio 2

✎ Coloque una cartulina en un lugar visible. Dibuje dos figuras representando una pareja (hombre y mujer). Entregue a cada alumno y alumna un marcador. Pida que cada uno(a) vaya añadiendo a cada una de las figuras, una pareja adicional con la cual tiene contacto sexual. Su grupo tendrá la oportunidad de ver gráficamente lo que sucedería si cada persona tuviera contacto sexual con un par de personas adicionales. Siga añadiendo parejas hasta llenar la cartulina.

✎ Al llenar la cartulina, pida a los alumnos(as) que sumen el total de personas contagiadas con el HIV/SIDA si la pareja original estuviera infectada. Ayúdeles a visualizar la seriedad de la epidemia, y la importancia de protegerse de los riesgos que conlleva la promiscuidad sexual.

¿Tienen algo que ver las drogas y el alcohol con el HIV/SIDA?

Las drogas y el alcohol colocan a la persona en mayor riesgo de contagio porque pueden alterar su forma de pensar y razonar. De esta forma usted está propenso a observar una conducta de riesgo para su salud.

Además, las personas que usan agujas para inyectarse sus drogas, corren un riesgo enorme de contraer el HIV/SIDA. Uno de los medios más comunes de transmisión del virus HIV es por agujas infectadas.

La iglesia cristiana no aprueba el uso de drogas por considerarlas una forma de abuso del cuerpo, que es un don de Dios. Pero si no se puede convencer a un joven de dejar las drogas, al menos comparta con él o ella la forma de prevenir la infección por agujas.

¿Qué puedo hacer si uso agujas?

Usted no debe compartir agujas con otras personas. Si usted usa o comparte una aguja, lávela cuatro veces con cloro y, después, cuatro veces con agua.

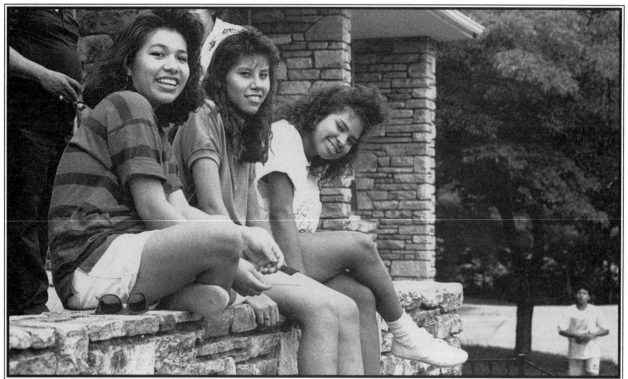

PHOTO BY SID DORRIS

Síntomas de la infección

Puede tener:

➤ Fiebre
➤ Fátiga
➤ Diarrea
➤ Erupciones en la piel
➤ Sudor nocturno
➤ Pérdida del apetito
➤ Glándulas linfáticas inflamadas
➤ Falta de resistencia a las infecciones
➤ Manchas blancas sarrosas en la boca
➤ Tos seca y falta de aliento
➤ Problemas con la memoria y los movimientos
➤ Manchas rojas o violeta en el cuerpo
➤ Pérdida de peso

No tener estos síntomas puede indicar que no tiene el HIV/SIDA. Pero recuerde que hay personas que no tienen síntomas al principio. Solamente haciéndose un examen de HIV puede usted asegurarse de no tener la infección.

La prueba del HIV

Hay dos reacciones muy comunes entre nuestra juventud (en adultos también) cuando se habla del HIV/SIDA: negación e inmovilidad. La negación puede hacer a una persona joven decir que no le va a suceder nada, que el HIV/SIDA es problema de otras personas. O puede hacerle pensar que es mejor no saber si tiene o no tiene HIV/SIDA. La negación es, no sólo peligrosa para la persona que observa dicha conducta, sino para las personas a las que puede contagiar. La persona que se inmoviliza ante la situación, siente tanto miedo, que no sabe que hacer. El miedo puede crear, además, odios y prejuicios contra las personas con SIDA.

Por las razones antes mencionadas, muchas personas jóvenes se niegan a seguir los consejos básicos que se sugieren. Además, pueden negarse a hacerse un examen para comprobar si tienen HIV+. Mientras mayor número de conductas de riesgo tiene una persona, más miedo puede sentir de conocer la verdad. Como líder de la juventud, usted puede tratar de ayudar a su grupo a actuar en forma responsable consigo mismos y con las demás personas.

Antes de hablar del examen del SIDA, explique al grupo cómo se desarollan los anticuerpos contra el virus de HIV. Generalmente se demora 6 a 12 semanas antes de que las defensas de nuestro cuerpo empiecen a producir anticuerpos. Este período se llama el período umbral. Durante este tiempo usted puede ser HIV+, pero sus anticuerpos no se han desarrollado y puede aparecer en la prueba como negativo. Usted debe esperar de 3 a 6 meses sin tener relaciones sexuales y sin compartir agujas para que su examen sea más preciso.

¿Quién debe examinarse?

➤ Personas que usan drogas y que comparten agujas
➤ Compañeros sexuales de personas adictas a drogas que comparten agujas
➤ Aquellos que tienen relaciones sexuales sin usar un condón

¿Por qué debo hacerme la prueba?

➤ Para asegurarse de que usted no tiene HIV/SIDA
➤ Para asegurarse de que usted no está pasando el virus del SIDA a otros
➤ Para poder mantenerse sano y saludable por más tiempo, si es que tiene el virus del SIDA

¿Dónde puedo examinarme?

Usted se puede examinar en el Departamento de Salud de su ciudad. Si el Departamento de Salud no hace el examen del SIDA, ellos le recomendarán otra agencia que esté cualificada para hacer el examen.

¿Cuál es la diferencia entre un examen anónimo y un examen confidencial?

Cuando una persona va a hacerse el examen del SIDA, le preguntan si desea un examen anónimo o confidencial. Muchos jóvenes no saben la diferencia.

Anónimo: Usted no da su nombre ni apellido. Le darán un numero de identificación a la hora del examen. Usted tiene que llevar el número a la oficina para obtener los resultados. En lugar de colocar su nombre, en el archivo se colocará un número.

Confidencial: Usted da su nombre y apellido. Esta forma de examinar es menos común hoy en día. Todavía existe la discriminación contra personas que tienen el SIDA, y muchas personas se sienten incómodas al usar este método de examen.

Nota: Todos los resultados de la prueba del SIDA, sean anónimos o confidenciales, son protegidos por la ley. Cualquier forma de injusticia se debe reportar.

¿Qué hago si mi amigo tiene el HIV/SIDA?

Sea como siempre lo fue. Una persona con SIDA necesita el cariño y la atención de sus seres queridos. Recuerde que usted no puede contraer el HIV/SIDA por estar cerca de alguien con el virus. Usted no se tiene que alejar o romper la amistad. El SIDA no se propaga por contacto casual.

Ejercicio 3

✎ Use el Ejercicio 1 nuevamente. Permita a sus alumnos y alumnas comprobar cuánto han aprendido por medio del programa.

Conclusión

Nuestra juventud cada a día más afectada por el virus que causa el SIDA (HIV+). Este virus no solamente destruye vidas, también destruye a la familia. La familia hispana siempre a sido unida, y la pérdida de un ser querido es muy dolorosa. Nuestro deber como hispanos es educar a la juventud para que difruten de una larga y duradera vida llena de salud, tal como Dios quiere para todos sus hijos e hijas.

Eliecel Rodríguez nació en Cuba. Vive en Connecticut donde hace estudios universitarios. Fue aprobado por la Cruz Raja como Instructor de HIV/SIDA en 1990. Trabajó como Director de educación sobre HIV/SIDA para jóvenes. Tiene planes de seguir la carrera de medicina.

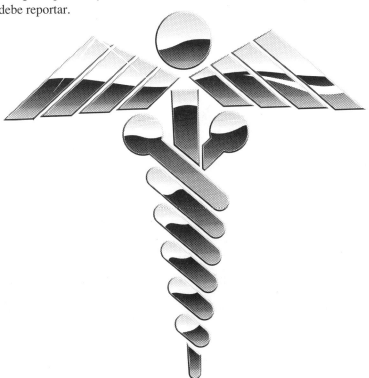

El SIDA y las emociones en la familia

Por Raúl R. Gómez

¿Qué tensiones emocionales confronta la persona que es diagnósticada con HIV/SIDA?

Ser diagnosticado con HIV+ o SIDA es un evento dramático, espantoso, y deprimente. Antes de la introducción de medicinas para combatir el HIV+/SIDA, no había esperanza de tratamiento. El diagnóstico de HIV+/SIDA significa enfrentarse a la posibilidad real y próxima de la muerte. Especialmente para la juventud diagnosticada con SIDA, esto significa olvidarse de nociones de inmortalidad y, repentinamente, tener que preocuparse por un futuro incierto y limitado.

Muchas pérdidas ocurren: pérdida física de función y salud, pérdida de ingresos debido a incapacidad física, pérdida de compañerismo y de sistemas de apoyo debido a ignorancia y prejuicio, entre otras cosas. En algunos casos se añade el rechazo por parte de la comunidad o de personas que temen ser contagiadas. Como consecuencia, puede surgir en la persona enferma un sentimiento de vacío personal, social y familiar.

El miedo al futuro, el miedo a la muerte, el temor al sufrimiento físico son reacciones posibles desde las primeras etapas de la enfermedad. Para una persona joven puede haber un choque entre su ilusión de inmortalidad (no se piensa mucho en la muerte en esa época de la vida) y la inminencia de la muerte. Muchos planes e ilusiones para el futuro deben cambiarse. Hay ajustes que hacer a causa de las pérdidas a las que se enfrenta el paciente.

La pérdida de salud física quiere decir que el individuo con SIDA gradualmente experimenta más dificultad al hacer deberes que antes hacía con facilidad. La fatiga disminuye sus actividades. Falta de apetito, pérdida de peso, diarrea, tos y fiebres hacen su efecto. Aún algunas medicinas recetadas al paciente pueden causarle problemas debilitantes tales como naúsea y anemia.

El enfermo con SIDA puede sentirse pesimista y perder la esperanza. Algunos pierden el ánimo completamente, dejan de tomar sus medicinas y dejan de ver al médico. El extremo puede ser la depresión severa, el aislamiento, y la pérdida del deseo de vivir al sufrir el dolor inaguantable del SIDA. Segun se acerca la muerte, el enfermo puede hacer decisiones sobre la prolongación artificial de la vida.

La pérdida de ingresos sucede en diferentes maneras. Algunas personas pierden su empleo simplemente a causa del diagnóstico. Las nuevas leyes sobre limitaciones físicas tal vez ayuden a reducir este tipo de discriminación,

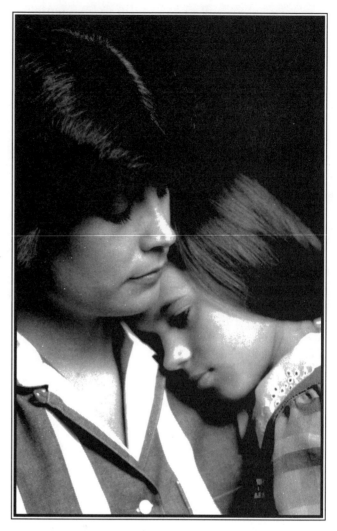

ya que el SIDA es considerado una limitación física. Debido a la fatiga y enfermedad, la persona tendrá que dedicar menos horas al trabajo, consiguiendo tiempo libre especial y por último, simplemente dejar de trabajar completamente. Al mismo tiempo, los gastos en medicamentos crecerán—no es raro que los gastos médicos aumenten a $500 por mes! Un período de siete días en el hospital puede ascender a más de $10,000. Otros obstáculos: falta de transportación a las clínicas, pérdida de trabajo por tener citas con el médico, problemas con el idioma. También los enfermos hispanos desconfían más de la comunidad medica debido a barreras culturales.

En el caso de una persona joven, puede resultarle difícil estudiar o seguir asistiendo a clases con regularidad. En algunos lugares las personas enfermas han experimentado el rechazo por parte de sus compañeros(as) de clase, de los padres de estos y hasta de las autoridades escolares. En algunos casos, el estudiante ha podido continuar en la escuela indefinidamente, pero en algunos otros ha tenido que seguir estudios en su casa. Se experimenta un rechazo social que resulta muy difícil para una persona de cualquier edad, pero en especial entre jóvenes.

¿Qué experimenta la familia del paciente?

La ansiedad acerca de todas las decisiones, planes, y cambios que deben hacerse, es común. Algunos enfermos deciden seguir participando activamente en las actividades regulares de su vida. Otros optan por pasividad y dejar que otros hagan las decisiones por ellos. En este último caso, es muy posible que los padres tengan que asumir responsabilidad en las decisiones.

A veces la familia de la persona enferma tiene sentimientos conflictivos o de rechazo al paciente. Estos sentimientos negativos pueden ser a causa de la desaprobación de algunos estilos de vida que pueden ser causa de la enfermedad. En otros casos se trata de sentimientos de vergüenza, de culpa o de temor ante el juicio de la comunidad en que viven. Debido al temor de contaminación, a algunas familias de personas enfermas se les ha dicho que se muden de la iglesia y de la vecindad. En caso de estos sentimientos negativos por parte de la familia, la soledad de la persona enferma puede ser mucho más profunda. Si no tienen otras personas con las cuales contar, la soledad añade dolor a los momentos de enfermedad por los que atraviesa el paciente.

Cuando una persona es diagnosticada con HIV+/SIDA ocurre una crisis con la cual la mayoría de las personas y familias hispanas no están preparadas a enfrentarse. Ira contra sí mismo, hacia el mundo, y aun contra Dios es una reacción frecuente a medida que la enfermedad avanza. Peor aún, el individuo con HIV+ puede negar que tiene SIDA, y negarse a buscar atención médica o a cambiar estilos de vida peligrosos.

¿Cuál debe ser la respuesta de la iglesia?

Una persona cristiana con SIDA puede encontrar que su fe religiosa es severamente puesta a prueba por el rechazo y prejuicio de otros cristianos. El enfermo puede culparse a sí mismo por su enfermedad, aún en aquellos casos en los cuales la persona no ha sido responsable (como en el caso de pacientes con hemofilia infectados con transfusiones de sangre).

Debido a que se sabe tan poco del SIDA, la enfermedad requiere comunicación muy cercana entre el paciente y su doctor. También el paciente y su familia necesitan aprender lo más posible acerca del HIV+/SIDA. Si el médico o el pastor(a) le explican a la familia y al paciente lo que pueden esperar en el proceso, estos tendrán mejor oportunidad de enfrentarse a la crisis.

Cuando la familia y amistades del enfermo conocen su diagnóstico, responden de maneras diversas. Algunos se aterrorizan y dejan de visitar o llamar al enfermo por temor al contagio. Algunos violarán la confidencialidad del paciente, compartiendo con otros el diagnóstico. También habrá juicios de la moral y rechazo del paciente. La familia cristiana que se encuentra con que uno de los suyos está contagiado con el SIDA, confronta muchas inseguridades, fuertes emociones, y conflictos religiosos. Lo importante es tratar con estas emociones y sentimientos abiertamente y no tratar de evadirlos.

La familia y amistades del paciente necesitan animarlo y respaldarlo hasta que pasen los tiempos de depresión y confusión. Frecuentemente un grupo de apoyo o consejería individual son vitales para ayudar a la persona con SIDA a manejar su situación. Ciudades como San Antonio, Texas y otras tienen agencias que proveen consejería gratis, servicios sociales, y recursos para el enfermo y su familia. Algunas agencias están dedicadas específicamente a clientes hispanos. Si desea mayor información sobre agencias en su comunidad, puede consultar la sección *Recursos en español* y *Where To Go For Help* en las páginas 95-96 y la portada interior de este recurso.

La respuesta de la iglesia a víctimas del SIDA debe ser una de compasión y de aceptación. El apoyo y consejo de la iglesia puede ayudar a la persona enferma y a la familia a mantenerse en fe y con fortaleza en medio de la crisis. Puede ayudar al paciente a poner su vida en paz, a prepararse para cada momento de la enfermedad, y a aceptar el futuro. Esto puede ser especialmente difícil para una persona joven. El reto es usar nuestra fe bíblica para que nos guíe a enfrentar con sabiduría problemas que no podemos resolver, y asuntos que no podemos comprender.

Para reflexión:

✎ Pida a varios alumnos(as) que preparen un drama para representar la reacción de una persona joven al recibir la noticia de que tiene HIV+. Esa persona joven debe darle a su familia la noticia sobre el diagnóstico. Use la información en el artículo como base para preparar el psicodrama.

Si su grupo está formado de personas muy jóvenes, usted y un grupo selecto de jóvenes pueden escribir el drama. Trate de ayudarles a entender los sentimientos de la persona que descubre que tiene HIV+/SIDA y las reacciones de las personas allegadas.

✎ Otra manera de estudiar el artículo es pedir a la clase que identifique algunas de sus reacciones respecto al SIDA. Divida al grupo en dos. Un grupo puede anotar en un papel todas las emociones que puede sentir una persona que recibe el diagnóstico de que tiene HIV+/SIDA. Deben tomar en cuenta las diferentes formas en que puede contagiarse la enfermedad. Otro grupo puede anotar las reacciones que puede tener la familia de una persona enferma, nuevamente considerando las diferentes formas en que puede suceder el contagio.

✎ Cuando terminen la discusión, un relator de cada grupo debe presentar un informe de las conclusiones a las que han llegado. Compare las conclusiones con la información del artículo. Añada los comentarios que completen la información.

Raúl R. Gómez M.D. es miembro de la Iglesia MetodistaUnida "La Trinidad" de San Antonio, Texas

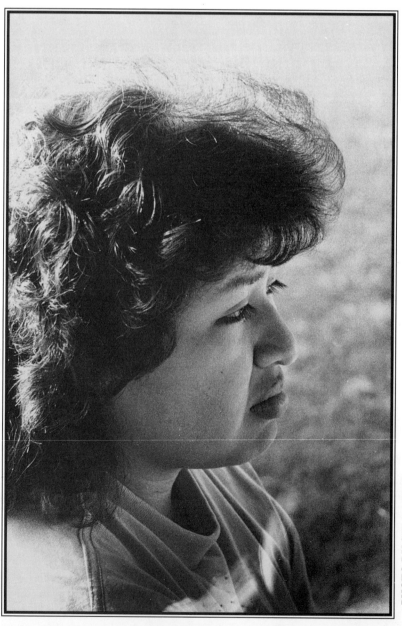

PHOTO BY SID DORRIS

La pastoral cristiana y la crisis del SIDA

por Héctor Ortíz

Este artículo tiene como propósito ofrecer a la juventud ideas sobre cómo ofrecer un testimonio cristiano frente a la crisis del SIDA.

Un proverbio chino indica que la palabra crisis presupone peligro y oportunidad. Cuando hablamos de la crisis del SIDA, vemos estas dos dimensiones presentes en la misma. Por un lado, la crisis del SIDA constituye una de las más formidables amenazas contra la vida humana. Por otro lado, representa la oportunidad de lograr muchas cosas; desde grandes descubrimientos científicos hasta un testimonio cristiano permeado por la misericordia hacia aquellos afectados por la condición.

El Síndrome de Inmunodeficiencia Adquirida (SIDA), constituye una enfermedad en la cual el sistema de inmunidad del cuerpo, el sistema de defensa contra las enfermedades, deja de funcionar. Cuando el sistema falla, una persona con SIDA típicamente desarrolla una variedad de enfermedades que ponen en peligro su vida y paulatinamente logran terminar con ésta. El SIDA es causado por el virus conocido como "virus de inmunodefiencia humana" o HIV.

Muchas personas piensan que los jóvenes no contraen el mismo, pero la experiencia nos indica que dichas personas están equivocadas. El SIDA puede afectar a cualquier persona, de cualquier edad, raza, u origen étnico. Cualquier persona que se exponga al virus HIV, el virus que causa el SIDA, tiene posibilidades de contraer la enfermedad. Hay lo que se llama comportamiento comprometedor o de riesgo con personas infectadas con el HIV, en el cual el contagio puede ocurrir con mayor probabilidad.

Desde el año 1981 hasta la otoño de 1992 se han diagnosticado con SIDA casi 40,000 personas entre las edades de 20 a 29 años en los EU. Un número significativo de éstas personas fueron infectadas con el virus del SIDA cuando eran adolescentes. Se sabe que una persona puede estar infectada por diez (10) años o más, antes de que las señales de la enfermedad aparezcan.

Muchos jóvenes tienen un comportamiento que aumenta el riesgo de ser infectados. Los comportamientos mediante el cual una persona joven puede infectarse con HIV son los siguientes:

➤ Teniendo relaciones sexuales, (ya sean vaginales, anales o tal vez orales) con una persona infectada.

➤ Compartiendo agujas o jerínguillas con una persona infectada.

➤ Las mujeres infectadas con el HIV pueden transmitir la infección a sus bebés durante el embarazo y el parto. En algunos casos pueden transmitir el HIV al dar el pecho a los bebés.

➤ Algunas personas han sido infectadas al recibir transfusiones de sangre, especialmente antes de 1985. (Desde el 1985 se comenzó el examen de laboratorio detallado de toda la sangre de donantes.)

Compartir información como las que se han estado presentando en este recurso es una de las formas más eficaces de combatir esta crisis. La juventud debe tener acceso a toda la información que les ayude a reconocer las situaciones de riesgo y a evitarlas.

Pero la información por sí sola, no es suficiente. Es necesario que la juventud reflexione también sobre la necesidad de tomar decisiones responsables e inteligentes acerca de cómo actuar de una manera saludable y evitar la infección por HIV.

Es importante que la juventud cristiana que lucha contra el SIDA vaya más allá del mero hecho de recibir información y adoptar decisiones inteligentes. Es necesario lograr una presencia cristiana más significativa en medio de esta crisis. Quisiera ofrecer varias ideas que nos ayuden a lograr una pastoral cristiana frente a la crisis del SIDA.

➤ Hablar de pastoral cristiana significa:
- presencia y testimonio cristiano en medio de la vida.
- gracia y misericordia para el enfermo (a) de SIDA.
- comprender que el SIDA es hoy equivalente a lo que fue la lepra en el pasado.
- reflexionar sobre cómo nuestro Señor Jesucristo ayudó a los leprosos de su época.

➤ La pastoral cristiana requiere:
- aproximación a la tarea llenos de misericordia.
- estar dispuestos a tocar a las personas enfermas tal como lo hizo Jesús.
- comprometernos a humanizar nuestra relación con los infectados por el virus.
- examinar nuestra conciencia para reconocer los prejuicios y miedos que el tema nos plantea.
- exige una oración penitencial y de perdón por la insensibilidad que muchas veces hemos demostrado.

➤ Hablar de una pastoral cristiana para enfrentar la crisis del SIDA exige:
- un entendimiento claro de la sexualidad humana a la luz del evangelio.
- una comprensión amplia de las implicaciones de dicho entendimiento sobre la sexualidad para una ética cristiana de la sexualidad.

➤ Ofrecer un testimonio cristiano permeado por la misericordia frente a la crisis del SIDA exige:
- • evitar la tendencia a adoptar posiciones farisaicas frente a issues controversiales.
- • evitar la tendencia a juzgar a los infectados como si fueran sólo seres faltos de fe o castigados por Dios.

En resumen, vivir una pastoral cristiana frente a la crisis del SIDA exige un compromiso de trabajar buscando prevenir la condición. Requiere involucrarse activamente en una pastoral de consolación y misericordia con todos aquellos que sufren de forma directa ó indirecta el flagelo del SIDA.

A esa pastoral cristiana, nuestro Señor Jesucristo nos invita hoy. Así nos ayude Dios.

Para la reflexión:

✎ La palabra crisis tiene dos significados en chino: peligro y oportunidad. Escriba la palabra crisis y sus dos significados en un papel grande o en una pizarra. Usando la técnica de torbellino de ideas, pida al grupo que considere la crisis del SIDA en ambos sentidos.

✤ ¿En qué sentido se trata de peligro?

✤ ¿En qué sentido es una oportunidad?

Este ejercicio se puede llevar a cabo antes de comenzar la discusión del artículo, para comprobar las actitudes y conocimientos del tema que tiene su grupo. Al terminar la discusión, pídales que consideren nuevamente el doble significado y evalúen sus respuestas iniciales. Pueden eliminar, añadir o corregir sus respuestas de acuerdo a los nuevos puntos de vista que hayan adquirido.

✎ Hay tres aspectos de la tarea pastoral acerca del SIDA que se sugiere tomar en cuenta: la juventud necesita información, la juventud necesita aprender a tomar decisiones éticas basadas en el Evangelio, la juventud necesita comprometerse a ayudar a otras personas. Divida al grupo en tres y asígnele un aspecto a cada uno. Pídales que evalúen lo que se está llevando a cabo en su grupo y en su congregación en estos tres aspectos y lo que puede hacerse. Cada grupo pequeño puede compartir con el grupo total las conclusiones de su discusión.

✎ En el artículo se mencionan una serie de características necesarias para desarrollar una presencia cristiana en medio de la crisis. Se le llama a esa presencia "pastoral cristiana". Tome una de las historias en este recurso (en inglés o en español), compártala con el grupo y analízela de acuerdo a los principios que sugiere el artículo.

✤ ¿De qué manera se puede convertir la situación en una oportunidad para la pastoral cristiana?

✎ ¿Qué dice la Biblia?:

✳ Estudien **Marcos 1:40-45**. Esta es la historia de un leproso, una persona a la cual la gente de la época de Jesús no se acercaba por temor al contagio.

✤ ¿Cuál fue la actitud de Jesús hacia este hombre?

✤ ¿Fue esa una actuación extraña por parte de Jesús o se portaba él siempre igual con los enfermos? Compare las respuestas del grupo con **Marcos 2:17**.

✳ Examinen la parábola en **Lucas 15:11-32**.

✤ ¿Cómo se describe a Dios en esa parábola?

✤ ¿Cómo se puede aplicar este mensaje a la pastoral cristiana?

Héctor Ortíz es ministro ordenado de la Iglesia Metodista de Puerto Rico. Pastorea la Iglesia Metodista Santísima Trinidad en San Juan, Puerto Rico. El Revdo. Ortíz es psicólogo clínico.

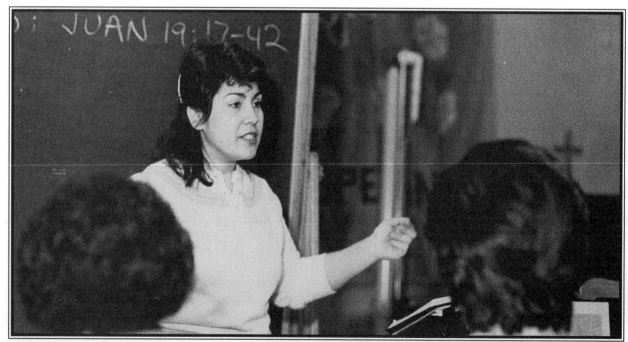

PHOTO BY SID DORRIS

Mis hermanos más pequeños

por Marta Sanfiel

Textos bíblicos:
1 Corintios 12:24b-26; Mateo 25:39-40

Propósitos:

➤ Ayudar a la juventud a comprender que no hay alternativa para la persona cristiana en particular o/y para la iglesia en general en cuanto a tomar amoroso cuidado del enfermo/a de SIDA. Al igual que cualquier otro ser humano en sufrimiento, el o ella, se convierte en nuestro hermano/a más pequeño/a, de quien habremos de rendir cuentas a Dios.

➤ Identificar, a través de las experiencias relatadas, las distintas formas en que la juventud de la iglesia puede prestar ayuda a los enfermos de SIDA y a sus familiares.

La llamada

La tarde era fría y lloviznosa. Trabajaba tranquilamente en mi oficina cuando el teléfono sonó. Al otro lado de la línea oí la voz alegre de una de las damas de la iglesia. Después de los saludos de costumbre me dijo: "Pastora, ¿sería usted capaz de ir a ministrarle a un enfermo de SIDA que se está muriendo en el hospital?"—"Por supuesto que sí"—repliqué. Me dió los detalles rápidamente. Era un joven hispano. Nunca había querido aceptar a Cristo como Señor de su vida. Ahora yacía moribundo en un hospital con el estigma de estar enfermo de SIDA, ser homosexual e hispano. Cuando terminé la conversación comenzaron las preguntas en mi mente: ¿"Que voy a decirle a ese joven?" "No tiene conexión con la iglesia, no quiere saber de Cristo y es homosexual. ¿Merece que me arriesgue a ir hasta él?" Las preguntas se convirtieron en diálogo con el Señor. La oración requería la dinámica de la respuesta inmediata, respuesta que no se hizo esperar: "Te daré palabras"—me respondió el Señor. Pero, "¿está mi lugar con un homosexual enfermo de SIDA?"—insisti, en mi afán de librarme de aquella misión a la cual temía, más que nada, por ser nueva y desconocida. Como el rumor de muchas aguas me llegó el mensaje de Cristo: "Estuve enfermo . . . y no me visitasteis . . . por cuanto lo hicisteis a uno de estos mis hermanos más pequeños, a mí lo hicisteis. . . apartaré a unos a mi derecha y a otros a mi izquierda . . ."

¡No había alternativa! ¡Tendría que ir!

La reflexión

Cuando Cristo nos habla de nuestra responsabilidad personal con los que sufren y entre los mismos menciona a los enfermos, no hace distinción en cuanto a qué tipo de dolencia deben padecer para servirles como se sirve al Señor mismo. No hay una palabra ni una frase que nos hable de distinciones entre los enfermos. Cuando nos habla de distinciones es al final del capítulo 25, en que se presenta el cuadro del día en que habrá de hacer separación entre los que sirvieron en su nombre, y los que se negaron a hacerlo o simplemente no se preocuparon por hacerlo.

La iglesia, como cuerpo de Cristo y la juventud cris-

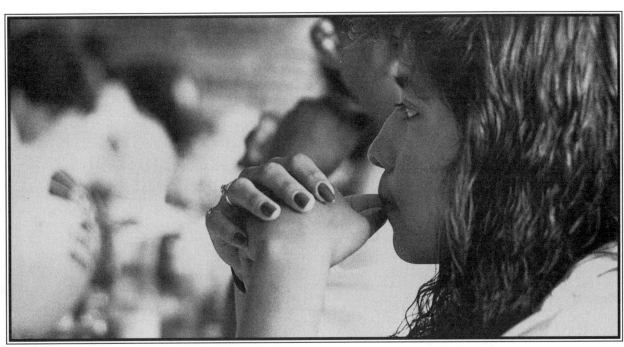

tiana como seguidora de Jesús está comprometida en una relación de cuidado hacia las personas enfermos. Este compromiso debe revelarse en acción y no limitarse a palabras y declaraciones.

Hay iglesias y personas cristianas que creen que una campaña de educación y algunas donaciones de dinero son suficientes para cumplir este compromiso de cuidar a las personas enfermas. Sin embargo, creo que el Señor demanda que nos involucremos personalmente con los "hermanos más pequeños".

El ministerio

Fue precisamente esa convicción la que me decidió a ir al hospital a ver a aquel joven. Nunca pude escuchar una palabra de sus labios. Ya no hablaba. Apenas entreabría los ojos de cuando en cuando. Durante las pocas semanas que le quedaron de vida todo lo que pude hacer fue ponerle mi mano sobre su frente y orar.

Sin embargo, conocí a su familia, sus amistades allegadas, algunos miembros del personal médico. A todos les hablé de Cristo. Siempre llegábamos a la misma conclusión: la ciencia había agotado sus recursos para salvar el cuerpo del enfermo. Ahora sólo quedaba rescatar su alma, y brindar apoyo espiritual y ayuda material a la familia. Finalmente el joven murió. Dirigí su servicio funeral y parte de la familia ha quedado para siempre en la iglesia.

Ahora bien, esa experiencia que acabo de compartir fue personal. La iglesia poco o casi nada tuvo que ver en el caso. Pero, ¿qué pasa cuando el enfermo llega a la iglesia y quiere ser parte de la congregación?

Otra situación

Había recién comenzado el culto de domingo cuando lo ví entrando por la puerta de la iglesia. El paso tambaleante, su rostro pálido, su cuerpo extremadamente delgado denunciaba su mal. Se sentó en la parte de atrás del santuario. Cuando hice la invitación a venir al altar a orar todos los que tuvieran una necesidad especial, el llegó. Allí, entre sollozos, me pidió que orara porque el Señor le sanara. Después del culto lo invité a que se quedara a tomar café. Aunque temeroso, aceptó. Ese fue el comienzo de otra oportunidad de ministerio con un enfermo de SIDA al que llamaré Tony.

Ese primer domingo la congregacion lo trató cordialmente pero con retraimiento. Una ancianita se me acercó y me dijo: "Pastora, tenga cuidado con las lágrimas de Tony, pueden ser muy peligrosas". Fue el comienzo de sus últimos quince meses de vida, y los primeros quince meses de vida de una congregación que se comprometió en el servicio a los que sufren.

Tony nos abrió las puertas de su casa para estudios bíblicos y allí asistimos aquellos que creíamos en el amor. Me pidió una oportunidad para cantar en la iglesia y se la dí. Poco a poco el miedo fue desapareciendo de

parte de los hermanos. Yo veía a Tony una vez por semana en mi oficina. Ahí aprendió el amor de Cristo y su perdón, y se entregó a El. A medida que el tiempo avanzaba, él se deterioraba más.

Comenzaron los hermanos a turnarse para llevarlo a las citas con el médico. Por fin se vió precisado a mandar a buscar a su madre. Fue la iglesia quien le proveyó transporte, quien la consoló. Luego llegó uno de sus hermanos carnales para atenderlo en sus últimos días. Se dio cuenta,

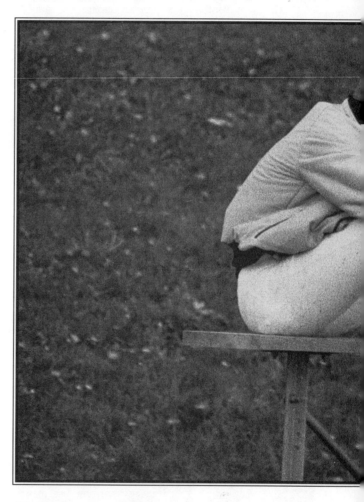

su hermano, del cambio en Tony. Le resultaba increíble el amor con que todos lo trataban. Una madrugada Tony se fue tranquilo y sonriente a vivir con el Señor.

Vino su familia inmediata y encontró que la única familia que Tony tenía en la ciudad era la iglesia. Su hermano pidió ir al edificio y conocer aquel lugar santo que había hecho tanto por su hermano.

El servicio memorial fue sencillo y estaban presentes sólo la familia de la carne y la de la fe. Todos sus parientes regresaron a sus pueblos. Sólo quedó la madre para recoger las cenizas, limpiar la casa, decidir qué hacer con las posesiones del muchacho. Fueron las damas de la iglesia las que acompañaron a su madre hasta que terminó, las que le ayudaron a limpiar, las que se quedaron a dormir con ella en la casa donde Tony había vivido y muerto. Antes de marcharse del pueblo me llamó y me dijo: "Jamás los olvidaré". Pero lo dijo en inglés porque Tony era norteamericano y asistía a la congregación anglo que yo pastoreaba; pero las damas que tanto ayudaron a Tony y a su mamá eran hispanas. Las dos congregaciones que se reunían en el mismo edificio se juntaron para servir al Señor, como espero que se junten para recibir la bienaventuranza en el día final.

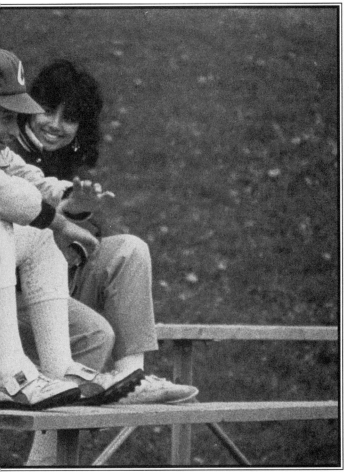

BY SKJOLD PHOTOGRAPHS

Si analizamos las historias que hemos hecho, podemos encontrar las diferentes formas en que una congregación o más de una, como sucedió con Tony, puede involucrarse en su compromiso de servir al Señor.

Consejos para el cuidado cristiano
➤ Aceptar a la persona enferma de SIDA como a cualquier otra persona enferma. Sin pasar juicios, reconocer el sufrimiento físico y espiritual por el que el o ella está pasando y tratar de aliviarlo.

➤ Hacerle saber que cualquier manera en que ellos o ellas quieran compartir sus fuerzas, talento y dinero con usted o su grupo serán aceptados.

➤ Demostrarles la disposición de ayudarles en sus necesidades materiales (llevarlos al médico, hacerles mandados, prepararles comida, llamar a sus familiares cuando hay una crisis y otras)

➤ Pedirle al pastor o la pastora que le asista con consejo pastoral y que le muestre el camino de la salvación.

➤ Ayudar en la reconciliación de la familia en cuanto sea posible. Hay casos en que algunos miembros de la familia se niegan a reconocer al enfermo y no quieren responder a su llamado. Otras veces hay viejas rencillas que mantienen a la familia desunida, aumentando el sufrimiento del enfermo. Somos llamados al ministerio de la reconciliación. Le sugerimos que busque la ayuda del pastor o pastora para estos casos.

➤ Estar presente en el funeral. Esto es un testimonio de gran valor para familias y amigos.

➤ Debido a que la enfermedad del SIDA se ha asociado con la práctica de la homosexualidad (aunque sabemos que puede ser contraído también por heterosexuales y a través de otras vías que no son el sexo) casi siempre el enfermo y la familia forman un núcleo aparte. La iglesia, representada por su juventud, tiene una oportunidad tremenda para ministrar a estas personas que se sienten tan desoladas, y hacerles sentir el amor de Cristo a través del amor a ellos.

¿Que puede hacer la juventud?
➤ Preparar un tablón de anuncios donde presentarle a la congregación la posibilidad de que un día alguno de sus miembros puede ser diagnosticado con el mal o alguna persona enferma puede empezar a asistir a la iglesia en su búsqueda del Señor.

➤ Organizar una conferencia sobre la enfermedad, brindando información al día, científica y en palabras que puedan ser claramente entendidas. Invitar a toda la membresía de la iglesia.

➤ Organizar un estudio bíblico basado en **Mateo 25** y otro en **1 de Corintios 12**. Relacionar los textos con la actitud cristiana hacia las personas enfermas.

➤ Organizar un grupo formado por personas de todas las edades para visitar uno de los centros que se dedica a cuidar personas enfermas de SIDA. Lléveles alguna ayuda en dinero u objetos de uso personal. Visite luego una de las salas de cáncer de un hospital y lléveles una ayuda similar.

➤ Reunir al grupo para discutir, a la luz de los estudios bíblicos y de sus visitas a los diferentes centros para enfermos, si ellos entienden que hay alguna diferencia entre nuestro compromiso como comunidad cristiana entre los enfermos, por razón de su diagnóstico.

Después de estos cinco pasos, creemos que la congregación estará mejor preparada para ejercer su misión entre los hermanos más pequeños.

Para reflexión:

✎ Se dice en el programa que Jesús no hizo distinción entre una persona enferma y otra. Todos los que fueron a Jesús fueron sanados. Escoja tres milagros de sanidad realizados por Jesús. Divida al grupo en tres y asígneles uno de los milagros para reflexión. Reflexionen como grupo en la actitud de Jesús cuando tuvo al enfermo o a la enferma delante de sí.

✤ ¿Reprendió él a la persona?

✤ ¿Le preguntó cómo se había enfermado?

✤ ¿Rechazó Jesús a alguna persona enferma o dió señales de que no quería ayudarle?

✎ En el programa se cita la parábola del juicio de las naciones como principio ético que debemos considerar al tratar a nuestro prójimo. En especial, la escritora dice que ese es su principio al ministrar a pacientes con HIV/SIDA.

✳ Lea y discuta el texto bíblico en **Mateo 25:31-46**.

✤ ¿Están de acuerdo con la interpretación del texto bíblico en el programa? ¿Por qué sí o por qué no? Si están en desacuerdo, ¿qué otro principio bíblico usarían?

✤ Si pensamos que Jesús está como una presencia viva en nuestro prójimo, ¿qué consecuencias tiene este hecho en nuestra actuación hacia una persona con HIV/SIDA?

✎ En forma de torbellino de ideas, pida al grupo que piense en lo que estarían dispuestos a hacer si creyeran que están sirviendo a Jesús al ayudar a un paciente.

✎ Reflexionen sobre la primera historia en el programa.

✤ La decisión estuvo basada en oración y en la reflexión sobre un texto bíblico que la pastora sintió que Jesús le inspiraba a considerar. ¿Qué principios usarían las personas jóvenes en su grupo para tomar una decisión como ésta?

✤ ¿Qué otros medios pueden ser usados para la toma de decisiones?

✤ Un prominente escritor cristiano sugiere que debemos considerar, además de la oración y la inspiración divina, la reflexión moral y el consejo de personas cristianas maduras. ¿Cuál sería la posición de sus jóvenes al respecto?

✤ Hubo una transformación en la vida de la familia del joven con SIDA, aunque no sabemos lo que ocurrió en la vida interior del joven mismo.

✤ ¿Creen que valió la pena el esfuerzo que hizo la pastora para ministrar a la vida de este joven enfermo?

✤ ¿Vale la pena ministrar, aunque no se vean resultados?

✤ El apoyo y la provisión de necesidades de las familias con pacientes de SIDA es muy importante. ¿De qué formas específicas puede ayudar la juventud?

✎ La segunda historia del programa sugiere que, aunque hay ayudas personales a personas enfermas con HIV/SIDA, la actitud de la congregación puede ser diferente.

✤ ¿Estuvo la actitud de la congregación guiada por un espíritu de amor cristiano o por pura tolerancia humana?

✤ ¿Creen que fueron muy liberales con el joven?

✎ Si tuvieran que participar en una discusión sobre la actitud de su congregación hacia un enfermo de HIV/SIDA, ¿qué posición tendrían? Este ejercicio puede ser hecho como un drama simulado, en el cual diferentes jóvenes hacen el papel de miembros de una junta de la iglesia.

✤ ¿En qué formas específicas puede ayudar la congregación a las familias de pacientes de SIDA?

✤ ¿De qué manera debe ayudar la iglesia a la comunidad a tomar actitudes diferentes hacia los pacientes de SIDA?

✎ Considere con el grupo la lista de consejos en las secciones *Consejos para el cuidado cristiano* y *¿Qué puede hacer la juventud?* Discuta los consejos y decida lo que la juventud de su congregación está en disposición de hacer por las personas con HIV/SIDA. Invítelos al compromiso.

Marta Sanfiel es original de Cuba. Es ministro ordenada de la Iglesia Metodista Unida. Pastorea dos congregaciones en New Orleans, Louisiana. Ha escrito en diversas ocasiones para Lecciones Cristianas y Lecciones Cristianas para jóvenes.

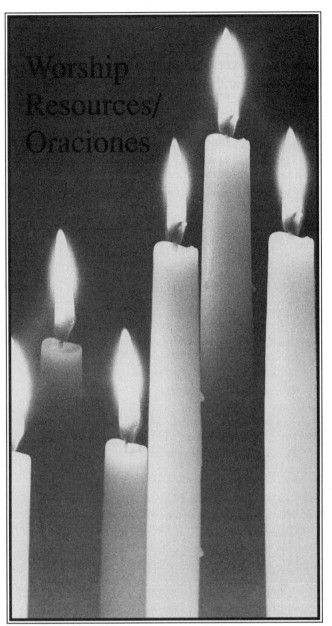

Worship
Resources/
Oraciones

Two thousand years ago, roofs were not as solid as most of ours today. They were made of mud and sticks, not asphalt or slate. Nonetheless, it still took some doing for a group of people to dig through a roof so a friend could receive Jesus' healing.

Their act might be difficult for us to understand today, not just because roofs have become more durable but because it is hard to imagine a group of people so anxious to be in Jesus' presence that they do something as drastic as digging through a roof.

These people teach us a powerful lesson about faithfulness. They feel so sure that Jesus will heal the man that they chance putting a hole in someone else's roof and interrupting Jesus' teaching.

They also provide an important model for HIV/AIDS ministry. In ministering to people with HIV/AIDS, situations arise that call us to go out of our way, "through the roof," so to speak. This is not to say that people with HIV/AIDS lay on mats, waiting for friends to carry them around. But there are times when barriers keep individuals with HIV/AIDS from receiving the care they need.

Facing these barriers alone sometimes leaves people with HIV/AIDS without hope. They need friends who are committed to removing obstacles that block them from what they need. The faithful actions of friends, caregivers, and loved ones can be one way people with HIV/AIDS feel Christ's presence and begin to experience healing.

————George R. Graham (*alive now!*)

Prepare Yourself to Encounter God

Through the Roof

When he returned to Capernaum after some days, it was reported that he [Jesus] was at home. So many gathered around that there was no longer room for them, not even in front of the door; and he was speaking the word to them. Then some people came, bringing to him a paralyzed man, carried by four of them. And when they could not bring him to Jesus because of the crowd, they removed the roof above him; and after having dug through it, they let down the mat on which the paralytic lay.
(**Mark 2:1-4**)

For Your Devotions

Worship Resources for HIV & AIDS Ministries by Patricia D. Brown and Adele K. Wilcox includes an introductory section, an Order of Sunday Worship, Using the Basic Pattern, and Personal Prayers. It is available from the Service Center, General Board of Global Ministries, 7820 Reading Road, Caller No. 1800, Cincinnati, OH 45222-1800, Stock number #1683. Cost is $2.50.

The theme for *alive now!*, January/February 1993 is "Spirituality for AIDS Ministries." *alive now!* is available from Upper Room Books, 1908 Grand Avenue, P.O. Box 189, Nashville, Tennessee 37202-0189. For orders and information, call (615) 340-7266.

Personal Prayers

❊ If only we could learn that the fulness of life is determined not so much by the length of our life as by the circumference of our heart and the depth of our love and understanding.

——-Arthur Louis McBride, 1955-1992 (*alive now!*)

❊ Lord God:

At times like this it seems so hard to trust in your infinite wisdom. We struggle against all odds to come to terms with such a diagnosis as has been given.

Pour out your love and comforting presence upon *Name* at this time. Give faith to bring our supplications for healing, for freedom from pain, and for strength for tomorrow to you.

We thank you for this day. Give us courage to respond to each day as it comes. In Christ's name we pray. **Amen.**

———*Worship Resources for HIV & AIDS Ministries*

❊ Spirit of God:

In this moment I am caught in fear and confusion.

I balance on the edge of my vulnerabilities; some imagined, some surprising, some painful.

Spirit of Truth:

In the still small voice I am aware of your nearness, which is strangely, mysteriously present to me; a smile in my friend's eyes, with bread and intimacy shared, in the silent moment alone.

Spirit of Life:

A deep longing brings me to your presence, and in the depths of my own holiness I cry that my spirit might be truly freed to be eased in my struggles, bold in staring down my terror, hopeful and free in my living, graceful in my life.

Spirit of Love:

Gentle my anger, quiet my desperation, soften my cynicism, soothe my fears.

Put me at peace and reconcile me with myself, and then with the people around me. **Amen.**

———*Worship Resources for HIV & AIDS Ministries*

Prayers for the Community

❊ AIDS Collect

Gracious God, you who bring to humankind your healing balm, making the pain and grief of life bearable, ease our suffering, give strength to our weakness, and deepen our compassion that we may reach out to our brothers and sisters in their illness and in their struggle against discrimination. In the name of the Creator, Redeemer, and Sustainer we pray. Amen.

——Ruth Sheets (*alive now!*)

❊ The Body of Christ Has AIDS

The Body of Christ has AIDS and we who are members are called to heal it.

Unto the least of these.

Feed the hungry—hungry for food, hungry for hope, hungry for love.

Clothe the naked—the naked body, the naked heart, the naked soul.

Heal the sick with love and care and hope.

The Body of Christ has AIDS and we are called to heal it.

We are not called to turn our backs. We are not called to cross to the other side. We are not called to blame the sick for their disease. We are called to heal.

Unto the least of these. Unto the sickest of these. Is it not we who will be dying if we do not?

——Peggy Jo Skill (*alive now!*)

❊ Almighty God, Lover and Creator:

I bring my prayers to you this day for persons anywhere who suffer from HIV infections and from the ravages of AIDS.

I confess Lord, that I do not understand a disease for which there appears to be no cure, for which there seems no hope for tomorrow.

All I can do is come to you and ask that you bring hope for those who are ill, especially for *Name(s).*

I pray for their families, their loved ones, and those who give them care.

When one whom I know is ill, Lord, I too suffer.

Keep me in close accord with those who are ill and bring me to action to help and advocate for them.

In the name of Jesus Christ I pray. **Amen.**

——(*Worship Resources for HIV & AIDS Ministries*)

❊ Holy One:

Today the reality of AIDS looms even larger because one of our own is ill,

It is easy, God, to want to ignore the sickness of someone else and to pretend that life is cheery for everyone.

Help me Lord to focus on another, to pray for my friend and companion, to remember ways to be of service, to give time to *his/her* caregiver, to make a meal, to sit and share.

God, you have placed me with a community of believers.

Yet I know that in the believing is also sharing, working together, and being the Christ for one another.

Help me to see the Christ in *Name.*

Enable me to be loving so that I might be Christ for another. **Amen.**

———*Worship Resources for HIV & AIDS Ministries*

Oraciones y ayudas litúrgicas

Letanía

Su grupo de jóvenes puede participar en algun culto de la iglesia o tener un culto propio para recordar a las personas enfermas con SIDA. Un culto especial de la iglesia sobre el tema del SIDA, o de los jóvenes invitando a otros grupos de la iglesia, puede ayudar a la congregación a pensar sobre el tema. Le sugerimos que permita que los jóvenes desarrollen su propio orden de culto. Esta letanía puede ser incorporada al programa.

Director(a): Dios de gracia y de vida, reconocemos tu presencia en medio de la humanidad que sufre.

Congregación: Te damos gracias porque nos muestras tu amor de muchas maneras cada día.

Director(a): Señor nuestro, te damos gracias porque en el éxodo de Egipto y en la cruz te identificaste con los sufrimientos de la humanidad.

Congregación: Te pedimos por los que hoy sufren diversas enfermedades, en especial de HIV positivo y de SIDA.

Director(a): Dios que nos das tu compañía, mira a las personas enfermas con SIDA que se sienten solas y abandonadas.

Congregación: Acompaña a cada una de estas personas enfermas, aclara sus mentes en medio de su confusión y sus preocupaciones, proveéles de la compañía que pueda llenar sus necesidades.

Director(a): Dios de la consolación, recordamos las familias de las personas enfermas de SIDA y sus sufrimientos.

Congregación: Ayuda a cada uno de los miembros de la familia a recibir consolación, dirección y fortaleza en medio de sus tristezas.

Director(a): Dios de la sabiduría, guía a los investigadores que tratan de encontrar una cura para el SIDA, así como al personal médico que atiende a las personas enfermas.

Congregación: Permite que sea posible encontrar la cura para el SIDA. Que con tu ayuda haya gozo en muchos hogares que hoy sufren por sus seres queridos enfermos.

Director(a): Dios de misericordia, concede doble dosis de paciencia, de amor y de inspiración divina a quienes se han dedicado a cuidar a las personas enfermas de SIDA.

Congregación: Permite que tengan la palabra sabia y el ánimo dispuesto para ser buena compañía de los pacientes cada día.

Director(a): Dios creador del universo, que nuestro mundo que lucha con la enfermedad, la muerte y el pecado pueda ser un día liberado con la liberacion final que has prometido en Cristo.

Congregación: Que como hijos e hijas vivamos haciendo tu voluntad y luchando por tu Reino.

Todos: Te damos gracias por tu presencia con cada uno de tus hijos e hijas cada día, así como por escuchar la oracion de tu pueblo.

Otras oraciones

Estas oraciones pueden ser usadas por los jóvenes si alguno de ellos visita a una persona enferma con SIDA. Según el estado físico o de ánimo de la persona enferma, pueden conversar un poco con el(la) paciente. Sugiera al joven o la joven que visite que no alargue su visita más de la cuenta. Es importante preguntar a la persona enferma cómo se siente ese día, y darle la oportunidad de que exprese sus sentimientos. Es importante, además, hablar de temas que ayuden a la persona enferma a sentirse animada.

❊ Dios de amor, te damos gracias porque tu nos has dado seguridad de que estás con nosotros todos los días de nuestra vida. Te pedimos que ayudes a este tu hijo(a) que se encuentra enfermo(a). Dale consuelo y fortaleza en medio de su necesidad. Permite que tenga la compañía de personas que les ayuden en las diferentes situaciones que tengan que enfrentar. Te lo pedimos en el nombre de Jesús. Amén.

❊ Dios que nos ayudas en nuestras tribulaciones, te pedimos que consueles a este tu hijo(a) en este momento de enfermedad. Es difícil tener paciencia o alegría cuando nos sentimos enfermos. Solamente la ayuda que viene con tu Espíritu Santo puede hacer que sintamos fuerzas para seguir esperando en tu ayuda. Te pedimos que seas el Consolador de este tu hijo(a) y que le ayudes a acercarse más a Ti en medio de la enfermedad. Por Jesucristo. Amén.

❊ Creador nuestro, nos acercamos a Ti confiando que tu nos escuchas. Este tu hijo(a) quiere rendir su vida a Ti porque cree que tu amor es importante en su vida. Te pedimos que seas la consolación de su vida y su fortaleza aún en los días más difíciles. Guía su vida por tus caminos. Por Jesucristo. Amén.

Just the Facts

➤ You may think that AIDS doesn't affect you, but if you don't know someone infected with HIV, chances are that you will soon.

"Our son was diagnosed with HIV in 1988. At that time he was suffering from these symptoms: a loss of vitality—he couldn't maintain his exercise program, he always felt tired and listless. He felt like he had the flu, and his immune system could not fight off constant infections."

Numbers (from Nashville CARES)

➤ The Centers for Disease Control **estimates** that 1 in every 100 adult males and 1 in every 800 female adults is infected with HIV.

➤ By the end of 1993, an estimated 390,000 to 480,000 people will have been diagnosed with AIDS.

➤ More Americans have already died from complications due to AIDS than were killed in the Korean, Vietnam, and Gulf Wars combined.

➤ 242,146 people nationwide have been diagnosed with AIDS. Of those diagnosed 141,223 have died.

➤ The World Health Organization predicts that the number of AIDS cases in the world will increase from an estimated 1.5 million in 1992 to 12-18 million by the year 2,000.

➤ An estimated 9-11 million people are currently infected worldwide.

➤ 75% of all cases worldwide are attributed to heterosexual transmission.

More Youth Numbers

Surveys have found that:

➤ As of fall 1992, more than 40,000 people ages 20-29 had been diagnosed with AIDS. Because a person can be infected for as long as 5 to 10 years before the signs of AIDS appear, a significant number of these young people would have been infected when they were teenagers.

"Two years after our son had been diagnosed with HIV he had lost 30 pounds. He felt like he never got enough sleep. When he did sleep he suffered from night sweats."

Symptoms*

➤ **Early symptoms**
   —fatigue
   —fever
   —diarrhea
   —enlarged lymph nodes
   —loss of appetite
   —night sweats
   —unexplained weight loss of 10 or more pounds
   —dry cough

"At eight months prior to his death, our son had no appetite. He had to be encouraged to eat small portions of food. Only a few things agreed with his stomach. He continued to lose weight and now at 6'1" he weighed only 140 pounds. He suffered from dysentery every day. His blood counts were below life levels."

➤ **Long term symptoms***
   —memory loss
   —indifference
   —loss of coordination
   —partial paralysis
   —mental disorder; damage to the brain and nervous system
   —dementia-forgetfulness, poor concentration
   —slowing down of movements, speech, and thinking
   —decreased alertness
   —loss of interest and pleasure in work, and most other activities
   —unpredictable or exaggerated changes in mood
   —several forms of cancer

"Four months prior to his death, our son was confined to a bed. The dysentery was so severe he had to stop using diapers. His bowels moved without him realizing it, 8-10 times a day into bed pans. At this time he also had to wear a bladder catheter. He was in constant, terrible pain. He took medications orally, rectally, and any way possible."

➤ Without treatment, half of HIV infected people will develop an AIDS-related illness within 10 years.

➤ HIV can be spread through sexual intercourse, from male to male, male to female, female to male, and in theory, from female to female.

➤ HIV can enter the body through cuts or sores in the skin or the moist lining of the vagina, penis, rectum, or even the mouth. *Some of these cuts or sores are so small you don't know they're there.*

"Four months prior to the death of our son, he was struck with shingles. The shingles robbed him of the use of one leg. He was hospitalized and two days later lost the use of his other leg. He was paralyzed from the waist down. The shingles got into his eyes and one side of his face. It was necessary to keep him in a dark room, and heavily medicated to ease the pain."

At Risk Checklist

There is evidence that HIV, the virus that causes AIDS, has been in the US at least since 1978. You may be at increased risk of infection if any of the following apply to you since 1978.

✤ Have you shared needles or syringes to inject drugs or steroids?

✤ If you are a male, have you had sex with other males?

✤ Have you had sex with someone who you know or suspect was infected with HIV?

✤ Have you had a sexually transmitted disease (STD)?

✤ Have you received blood transfusions or blood products between 1978 and 1985?

✤ Have you had sex with someone who would answer yes to any of the above questions? If you answer yes to any of the above questions, you should definitely seek counseling and testing.

➤ If you have had sex with someone and you didn't know their risk behavior, or you have had many sexual partners in the last ten years, then you have increased the chances that you might be infected with HIV.

➤ The only sure way to avoid infection through sex is to abstain from sexual intercourse or engage in sexual intercourse only with someone who is not infected and only has sex with you.

"Eighteen months prior his death, our son continued to loose weight. He still had an appetite, but food nauseated him. He had difficulty concentrating. He developed Kaposi's Sarcoma. These skin spots grew from the size of a dime to the size of a silver dollar. A nagging cough made it necessary for him to undergo breathing treatments at a local hospital."

How Not to Get Infected

➤ You won't get HIV through everyday contact with infected people at school, work, home, or anywhere else.

➤ You won't get HIV from clothes, phones, or toilet seats.

➤ You cannot get HIV from eating food prepared by an infected person.

➤ You won't get HIV from a mosquito bite. You won't get it from bedbugs, lice, flies, or other insects, either.

➤ You won't get HIV from sweat or tears.

➤ You won't get HIV from a simple kiss. Most scientists agree that although transmission of HIV through deep or prolonged kissing may be possible, it would be unlikely.

"Our son had TB of the bone, respiratory difficulties, severe bedsores, and was too weak even to turn over in bed. He couldn't sit up in bed because the bone pain was so severe. At four weeks prior to his death, he had Kaposi's Sarcoma sores on his nose, cheek, shoulder, arm, and back."

Why Seek Counseling and Testing

➤ Knowing whether you are HIV positive would alert you to your need to seek medical care to prevent or delay life-threatening illness.

➤ If you find out you are infected, knowing your result would help you protect your sexual partner(s) from infection and illness. If they are not infected, you can avoid infecting them.

➤ A negative test is not conclusive. If you have been infected with the virus recently, a negative test may mean that your body might not have had time to develop antibodies against the AIDS virus.

"During his last weeks our son was jumpy, anxious, and fearful. His nerves were destroyed. In the last three weeks he was totally blind."

Where to Go for Counseling and Testing

Depending on the area where you live, there are different counseling and testing places from which to choose. When you are making your choice, you want to consider these factors:

➤ If you have been to a particular place for health care, you may feel comfortable with the staff who will counsel you and offer you testing.

➤ If the center can provide immune system monitoring and medical care if you are infected with HIV, it might speed up the beginning of your medical treatment.

➤ Some counseling and testing centers offer special features. For instance, if you use drugs, you can receive counseling, testing, and help for addiction at a drug treatment facility.

Economics of AIDS

➤ Being infected with HIV is not only a health matter. It raises financial issues as well. One of these issues is insurance. Your ability to pay for health care can affect your access to monitoring and treatment. If you do not have health insurance or if you depend upon Medicaid, you may need special assistance to get treatment.

➤ Many insurance companies will not cover persons who have tested positive with HIV.

> "Our son was able to work up until eight months prior to his death. At that time he suffered from extreme fatigue and could only be up and about a few hours each day."

➤ A CDC study estimates the lifetime costs of treatment per AIDS patient in the United States ranges from $60,000 to $90,000.*

➤ Annual cost of AZT (azidothymidine or zidovudine) therapy is approximately $3470.00 (this information is per US FDA recommendation).*

> "Our son suffered severe headaches from taking AZT. As a result he took only two a day instead of the recommended dosage of twelve a day."

➤ Possible side effects of AZT include:*
   —anemia
   —nausea

Social Issues

➤ Some people who do not understand AIDS may avoid persons who they know are infected with HIV. Some people who are infected have been targets of discrimination in employment, housing, and insurance. Some have been deeply hurt by the reactions of friends and family members.

➤ You can show emotional support for an infected friend, associate, or acquaintance by trying one of the following:

✎ **Encourage the person with AIDS to become involved in his or her own care, set a schedule, and make decisions whenever possible.**
These actions will provide a sense of independence and control.

✎ **Don't avoid the person with AIDS.**
Include him or her in activities whenever possible. You don't always have to talk. Your company can be more important than your words. Just having you there while reading or watching television may be appreciated.

✎ **Don't be afraid to discuss the disease.**
Often, people with AIDS need to talk about it to work out in their own mind what is happening.

✎ **Most importantly, don't be afraid to touch a person with AIDS.**
Holding a hand, giving a hug, or giving a back rub can greatly raise the person's spirits. However, be sensitive to people who do not wish to accept physical closeness.

Caretaker Dos and Don'ts

Most people with AIDS can lead an active life for long periods of time. In fact, most of the time a person with AIDS does not need to be in a hospital. A person with AIDS often recovers from AIDS-related illnesses more quickly and comfortably at home with the support of friends and loved ones. Also, home care can help reduce the stress and cost of hospitalization.

✎ Do wear gloves if you have contact with blood or blood-tinged body fluids. If you clean up articles soiled with urine, feces, or vomit, wear gloves to avoid **other** germs. If disposable gloves are used, throw them away after one use. Household gloves can be reused if they are cleaned and disinfected after each use.
✎ Do wash your hands with soap and water after any hand contact with blood, even if gloves are worn.
✎ Do take the same precautions when vaginal secretions and semen are present.
✎ If you have cuts, sores, or breaks on exposed skin, cover them with a bandage.
✎ Do handle medication needles carefully.
✎ Do not ignore your own needs. Arrange for backup help so you can have some free time occasionally. Unless you take care of yourself, you will not have the inner resources to care for the person with AIDS.

> "Sixteen weeks before his death, our son was so deeply depressed and full of fear we never left him alone. During these last weeks, tender loving care was given round-the-clock by professionals, his family, and close friends."

AIDS Q&A
If somebody in my class at school has AIDS, am I likely to get it too?
➤ No. HIV is transmitted by sexual intercourse, needle sharing, or infected blood. It can also be given by an infected mother to her baby during pregnancy, birth, or breast-feeding.
➤ People infected with HIV cannot pass the virus to others through ordinary activities of young people in school.
➤ You will not become infected with HIV just by attending school with someone who is infected or who has AIDS.

Can I become infected with HIV from "French" kissing?
➤ Not likely. HIV occasionally can be found in saliva, but in very low concentrations—so low that scientists believe it is virtually impossible to transmit infection by deep kissing.
➤ The possibility exists that cuts or sores in the mouth

may provide direct access for HIV to enter the bloodstream during prolonged deep kissing. Still, most scientists agree that it would take a great deal of saliva to transmit the virus this way.

➤ There has never been a single case documented in which HIV was transmitted by kissing.

➤ **Scientists, however, cannot absolutely rule out the possibility of transmission during prolonged deep kissing.**

Can I become infected with HIV from oral intercourse?

➤ It may be possible.

➤ Oral intercourse often involves semen, vaginal secretions, or blood-fluids that can contain HIV.

➤ HIV is transmitted by the introduction of infected semen, vaginal secretions, or blood into another person's bloodstream.

➤ During oral intercourse, the virus might be able to enter the bloodstream through tiny cuts or sores in the mouth.

As long as I use a condom during sexual intercourse, I won't get AIDS, right?

➤ Far from being foolproof, condoms may break during intercourse.

➤ Condoms have been shown to help prevent HIV infection and other sexually transmitted diseases. Condoms in combination with a spermicide are the best preventive measure against the AIDS virus besides not having sex.

➤ You have to use them properly. And you have to use them every time you have sex—vaginal, anal, and oral.

➤ The only sure way to avoid infection through sex is to abstain from sexual intercourse, or engage in sexual intercourse only with someone who is not infected.

My friend has anal intercourse with her boyfriend so that she won't get pregnant. She won't get AIDS from doing that, right?

➤ Wrong. Anal intercourse with an infected partner is one of the ways HIV has been most frequently transmitted.

➤ Whether you are male or female, anal intercourse with an infected person is very risky.

If I have never used intravenous drugs and have had sexual intercourse only with a person of the opposite sex, could I have become infected with HIV?

➤ Yes. HIV does not discriminate. You do not have to be homosexual or an intravenous drug user to become infected.

➤ Both males and females can become infected and transmit the infection to another person through intercourse.

➤ If a previous sexual partner was infected, you may be infected as well.

Is it possible to become infected with HIV by donating blood?

➤ No. There is absolutely no risk of HIV infection from donating blood.

➤ Blood donation centers use a new, sterile needle for each donation.

Can I become infected with HIV from a toilet seat or other object I routinely use?

➤ No. HIV does not live on toilet seats, or other everyday objects, even those on which body fluids may sometimes be found. Other examples of everyday objects are doorknobs, phones, and drinking fountains.

A friend of mine told me that as long as I am taking birth control pills, I will never get AIDS. Is this true?

➤ No. Birth control pills do not protect against HIV.

➤ You can become infected with HIV while you are taking birth control pills.

➤ Even if you are taking the pill, you should use a condom and spermicide if you plan to have sex with someone whom you do not know to be uninfected.

What do I do if I think I am infected with HIV?

➤ Talk to someone about getting an HIV test that will determine if you are infected. That person might be a parent, doctor, or someone who works at an AIDS counseling and testing center.

➤ Call the National AIDS Hotline (1-800-342-AIDS) to find out where you can go in your area to get counseling about an HIV test. You don't have to give your name, and the call is free. You can also call your state or local health department. The number is under "Health Department" in the Government section of your telephone book.

➤ Your doctor may advise you to be counseled and tested if you have hemophilia or have received a blood transfusion between 1978 and 1985.

> "Our son died peacefully at 4 A.M. on January 31, 1992 a few days past his thirty-third birthday."

• Information in tint blocks courtesy of a family touched by AIDS.
• "Numbers (from Nashville CARES)" from Nashville CARES, 700 Craighead St., Nashville, TN 37204.
• Information marked with (*) provided by Centers for Disease Control, National AIDS Information Clearinghouse, P.O. Box 6003, Rockville, MD 20850.
• All other information quoted from CDC.

Solamente los hechos

➤ "Usted puede pensar que el SIDA no le afecta a usted; pero si no conoce a nadie con SIDA, las posibilidades son que llegue a conocer a alguien pronto."

Estadísticas

➤ El Centro para Control de Enfermedades estima que 1 de cada 100 varones adultos y 1 de cada 800 mujeres adultas estan infectados con HIV.

➤ Para finales de 1993, se estima que entre 390,000 y 480,000 personas serán diagnosticadas con SIDA.

➤ Más norteamericanos han muerto por complicaciones relacionadas con el SIDA que los muertos en Corea, Vietnam y la guerra del Golfo juntas.

➤ En los Estados Unidos 242,146 personas han sido diaguosticadas con SIDA. De estas un 141,223 han muerto.

➤ La Organización Mundial de la Salud anticipa que el número de casos de SIDA en el mundo aumentará de unos 1.5 millones en 1992 a entre 12 y 18 millones para el año 200.

➤ Se estima que hay entre 9 y 11 millones de personas infectadas con SIDA en el mundo.

➤ Un 75% de los casos en el mundo se atribuyen a transmisión heterosexual.

Síntomas tempranas

-fatiga
-fiebre
-diarrea
-nódulos linfáticos agrandados
-falta de apetito
-sudores nocturnos
-pérdidas inexplicables de peso de 10 libras o más
-tos seca

A largo plazo

-pérdida de memoria
-indiferencia
-pérdida de coordinación
-parálisis parcial
-desorden mental; daños al cerebro y al sistema nervioso
-demencia, olvido, concentración pobre
-movimientos, habla y pensamiento cada vez más lentos
-disminución en la energía
-pérdida de interés y de disfrute del trabajo, y otras actividades
-cambios impredescibles o exagerados de humor
-ciertos tipos de cáncer

➤ Sin tratamiento, la mitad de las personas infectadas con HIV desarrollarán enfermedades relacionadas con el SIDA dentro de los siguientes 10 años.

➤ Usted puede ser infectado(a) con HIV en dos formas principalmente:

➤ Por contacto sexual- anal, vaginal u oral- con una persona infectada.

➤ Por compartir agujas o jeringuillas con una persona infectada.

➤ El HIV puede propagarse a través del contacto sexual, de hombre a hombre, de hombre a mujer, de mujer a hombre y, en teoría, de mujer a mujer.

➤ El HIV puede infectar su cuerpo a través de cortaduras o lesiones en la piel, en la paredes vaginales, en el pene, en el recto, o en la boca. Algunas de estas cortaduras o lesiones son tan pequeñas que usted no sabe que las tiene.

➤ La única forma segura de evitar la infección a través del sexo es absteniéndose de contacto sexual o teniendo este sólo con una persona no infectada y que sólo tiene contacto sexual con usted.

La lista de riesgo

Hay evidencia de que el HIV, el virus que causa el SIDA, ha estado en los Estados Unidos al menos desde el 1978. Usted puede estar entre las personas con alto riesgo de infección si ha participado en alguna de estas actividades después de 1978.

✤ ¿Ha compartido agujas o jeringuillas para inyectarse drogas o esteroides?

✤ ¿Si es varón, ha tenido contacto sexual con otros varones?

✤ ¿Ha tenido contacto sexual con alguna persona que usted sospecha que está infectada con HIV?

✤ ¿Ha tenido una enfermedad transmisible sexualmente?

✤ ¿Ha recibido transfusiones de sangre entre 1978 y 1985?

✤ ¿Ha tenido contacto sexual con alguna persona que puede contestar afirmativamente a cualquiera de las preguntas anteriores? Si puede contestar afirmativamente a alguna de las preguntas anteriores, usted debe buscar consejo y examinarse, sin lugar a dudas.

✤ Si usted ha tenido contacto sexual con alguien y no ha estado consciente de su conducta peligrosa, o si ha tenido múltiples parejas sexuales en los últimos 10 años, entonces usted ha aumentado las posibilidades de estar infectado(a) con HIV.

No hay contagio si

➤ No va a infectarse con HIV por tener contacto con personas infectadas en la escuela, en el trabajo, en el hogar o en cualquier otro lugar.

➤ No va a infectarse al contacto con ropas, teléfonos o asientos de inodoro.

➤ No va a infectarse por comer alimentos preparados por una persona infectada.

➤ No va a infectarse por picadas de mosquito, de chinches, de piojos, de moscas o de otros insectos.

➤ No va a infectarse con sudor o con lágrimas de una persona infectada.

➤ No va a infectarse por un simple beso. La mayoría de los científicos están de acuerdo en que, aunque la transmisión del HIV a causa de besos profundos o prolongados es posible, no es probable.

Razones para buscar consejo y para examinarse

➤ El saber que tiene HIV le advierte sobre la necesidad de procurar tratamiento médico que prevenga o dilate la mortalidad. El resultado de su examen (positivo o negativo) también puede ayudar a su médico a determinar la causa y el mejor tratamiento de enfermedades que pudiera tener ahora o en el futuro. Por ejemplo, una persona HIV positiva, recibe un tratamiento para tuberculosis y sífilis diferente al que recibe una persona con HIV negativo.

➤ Si descubre que está infectado, este conocimiento puede ayudarle a proteger de la infección y de la enfermedad a su(s) compañero(s) o compañera(s) sexual. Si esa persona no está infectada, usted puede protegerles de infección.

➤ El conocer los resultados puede ayudarle a decidir si hay seguridad o no al tener un bebé.

➤ El saber el resultado de la prueba, aun si hubiera infección (un resultado positivo), puede ser menos inquietante para algunas personas que la ansiedad ante la posibilidad de estar infectado(a) y no saberlo. Si su resultado es negativo, puede tomar precauciones para evitar ser infectado(a) en el futuro.

➤ Un resultado negativo no cierra el caso. Si ha sido infectado(a) recientemente por el virus, un resultado negativo puede significar unicamente que su cuerpo no ha tenido tiempo para desarrollar los anticuerpos contra el virus que produce el SIDA.

La decisión sobre a dónde ir para recibir consejo y pruebas

Dependiendo del área del país donde usted viva, hay diferentes centros para consejería y pruebas. Sus alternativas pueden incluir centros para pruebas de HIV sostenidos con fondos públicos, clínicas de salud de la comunidad, clínicas de enfermedades sexualmente transmisibles, clínicas de planificación familiar, facilidades para el tratamiento de adicción a drogas, clínicas de tuberculosis, y oficinas de médicos. Cuando vaya a decidir puede tomar en cuenta los siguientes factores:

➤ Si ha estado en alguno de estos centros para tratamiento por alguna otra condición, puede sentirse cómodo(a) con el personal disponible para aconsejarle y para hacerle la prueba.

➤ Si el centro ofrece seguimiento médico en caso de estar infectado(a) con HIV, podría acelerarse el comienzo de su tratamiento.

➤ Algunos centros de consejo y tratamiento ofrecen servicios especiales. Por ejemplo, si usa drogas, puede recibir consejería, pruebas y ayuda para superar la adicción si el lugar donde se hace la prueba es una facilidad para tratamiento de la adicción a drogas.

Asuntos ecónomicos relacionados con el SIDA

➤ La infección por HIV no es sólo un asunto de salud. Tiene implicaciones sociales y financieras. Uno de los asuntos relacionados son los seguros. La habilidad que tenga la persona para pagar un seguro de salud puede afectar el acceso al tratamiento. Si la persona no tiene seguro de salud o si depende de Medicaid, puede necesitar ayuda económica para recibir tratamiento.

➤ Muchas compañías de seguro no ofrecen cubiertas para personas que han tenido resultados de HIV positivos.

➤ El costo anual del tratamiento AZT (Asidothymidine o Zidovudine) es de aproximadamente $3,470.00.

➤ Un estudio estima que el costo de tratamiento de un paciente de SIDA en los Estados Unidos puede ser entre $60,000 y $90,000.

Implicaciones sociales

➤ Algunas personas que no conocen sobre el SIDA pueden tratar de evitar a personas que ellos saben que están infectados con HIV. Algunas personas infectadas han sido víctimas de discriminación en empleos, vivienda y seguros. Algunos se han sentido heridos profundamente por las reacciones de amistades y de miembros de la familia. Si descubre que está infectado(a), debe prepararse para enfrentarse a reacciones desagradables.

➤ Usted puede dar apoyo emocional a amistades, compañeros(as) de oficina o personas relacionadas en alguna de las siguientes formas:

➤ Anime a la persona a encargarse de su cuidado personal, a tener un horario de actividades y a tomar sus propias decisiones siempre que sea posible. Estas actividades le pueden proveer a la persona un sentimiento de control y de independencia.

➤ No evite a la persona con SIDA. Incluya a esa persona en cuantas actividades sean posibles. No es necesario hablar. Su compañía puede ser más importante que sus palabras. El tener su compañía mientras lee o ve televisión puede ser muy apreciada por la persona enferma. Permita este tiempo quieto. Esa persona puede estar experimentando ira, frustración, depresión y muchas otras emociones.

➤ No tenga temor de discutir la enfermedad. A menudo, las personas con SIDA necesitan hablar sobre su enfermedad para poder procesar lo que está ocurriendo en su mente. Ofrézcále a la persona el conseguirle alguna ayuda profesional de consejería, si la persona lo desea. Permita que los médicos, las enfermeras(os) y los trabajadores sociales conozcan su relación con la persona enferma.

➤ Más importante aún, no tema tocar a una persona con SIDA. Tomar la mano, abrazar o dar un masaje en la espalda puede levantar el ánimo de la persona enferma. A la misma vez, respete el deseo de algunas personas que prefieren no aceptar ese contacto físico.

Números

➤ La Organización Mundial de la Salud anticipa que el número de casos de SIDA en el mundo aumentará de 1.5 millones en 1992 a entre 12 a 18 millones en el año 2000.

➤ Se estima que hay alrededor de 9 a 11 millones de personas infectadas en el mundo entero.

➤ Un 75% de los casos en el mundo se atribuyen al contacto heterosexual.

➤ Desde el otoño de 1992, más de 40,000 personas entre las edades de 20-29 años han sido diagnosticados con SIDA. Debido a que una persona puede estar infectada por 10 años o más antes de que las señales del SIDA aparezcan, un número significativo de estas personas jóvenes pueden haber sido infectados cuando eran adolescentes.

Recomendaciones para los encargados de pacientes

Muchos pacientes de SIDA pueden llevar una vida normal por largos períodos de tiempo. De hecho, la persona con SIDA permanece fuera del hospital la mayor parte del tiempo. Una persona con SIDA se recupera mejor y más rápidamente de enfermedades relacionadas con su condición cuando está en su casa bajo el cuidado y el sostén de amistades y seres queridos. Además, el cuidado en el hogar puede ayudar a reducir la tensión y el costo de la hospitalización.

➤ Use guantes si está en contacto con la sangre o con fluídos del cuerpo teñidos con sangre. Si limpia artículos llenos de orina, heces fecales o vómitos, use guantes para evitar los gérmenes, aunque no se hayan observado infecciones con HIV a través de dicho contacto. Si usa guantes desechables, elimínelos después de usarlos una vez. Los guantes caseros pueden usarse más de una vez si los limpia y desinfecta después de cada uso.

➤ Lávese las manos con jabón y agua después de cualquier contacto de sus manos con sangre, aún cuando use guantes.

➤ Si hay grandes cantidades de sangre, use una bata o delantal para prevenir que sus ropas se ensucien.

➤ Tome las mismas precauciones si hay secreciones vaginales o semen.

➤ Si tiene cortaduras o lesiones en la piel expuesta, cúbralas con un vendaje.

➤ Maneje las agujas hipodérmicas con mucho cuidado.

➤ No ignore sus propias necesidades. Haga arreglos para que alguien le sustituya de modo que pueda tener un tiempo libre de vez en cuando. A menos que usted se cuide a sí mismo(a), usted no tendrá los recursos interiores necesarios para cuidar a una persona enferma de SIDA.

Preguntas y respuestas sobre el SIDA

¿Si alguien en mi clase tiene SIDA, tengo posibilidades de contagiarme?

➤ No. El HIV se transmite por medio del contacto sexual, por compartir agujas o por transfusiones de sangre infectada. Puede también contagiarse al bebé durante el período de parto, de nacimiento o de lactancia (aunque esta posibilidad es rara) si la madre está infectada.

➤ Las personas infectadas con HIV no pueden transmitir el virus a otras personas a través de las actividades ordinarias de la gente joven en la escuela.

➤ No vas a infectarte con HIV sólo por asistir a una escuela donde alguien esté infectado con HIV o porque tenga SIDA.

¿Me podré infectar con HIV si beso a alguien con un beso profundo?

➤ No es probable que suceda. El HIV a veces puede encontrarse en la saliva, pero en concentraciones tan pequeñas que los científicos creen que es virtualmente imposible transmitir el virus a través del beso profundo.

➤ Existe la posibilidad de que las cortaduras o lesiones en la boca puedan brindar un acceso directo del HIV a la corriente sanguínea durante un beso prolongado. Aún así, la mayoría de los científicos están de acuerdo en que se requiere una gran cantidad de saliva para que el virus se transmita de esa manera.

➤ No hay ningun caso documentado en el cual el HIV se transmita por medio del beso.

➤ Los científicos, sin embargo, no pueden eliminar por completo la posibilidad de transmisión a través del beso prolongado profundo.

¿Puedo ser infectado(a) con HIV por tener contacto sexual en forma oral?

➤ Esto es posible.

➤ El contacto sexual en forma oral involucra semen, secreciones vaginales y otros fluídos sanguíneos que pueden contener HIV.

➤ El HIV se transmite por la introducción de semen infectado, secreciones vaginales o sangre en la corriente sanguínea de otra persona.

➤ Durante el contacto sexual en forma oral, el virus puede entrar a la corriente sanguínea a través de cortaduras leves o de lesiones en la boca.

Si uso condones durante el acto sexual, ¿ no me va a dar el SIDA, verdad?

➤ Los condones pueden romperse durante el acto sexual, por lo cual no son 100% seguros.

➤ Se ha comprobado que los condones pueden ayudar a prevenir la infección con HIV y otras enfermedades sexualmente transmisibles. El uso de condones, en combinación con el espermicida, es una de las medidas más efectivas para prevenir el contagio con el virus de SIDA, aparte de la abstinencia sexual.

➤ Tiene que usar los condones en forma apropiada para que estos sean efectivos. Y tiene que usarlos cada vez que tenga contacto sexual, sea este vaginal, anal u oral.

➤ La única manera segura para evitar el contagio a través del sexo es absteniéndose de contacto sexual, o manteniendo relaciones sólo con una persona que no esté infectada.

Mi amiga tiene contacto sexual con su novio en forma anal para evitar un embarazo. A ella no le va a dar SIDA si tiene relaciones de esa manera, verdad?

➤ Falso. El contacto sexual anal con un compañero infectado es una de las manera en que se transmite el HIV más frecuentemente.

➤ Aunque usted sea hombre o mujer, el contacto sexual en forma anal con una persona infectada es muy arriesgado.

¿Si yo nunca he usado drogas intravenosas y sólo he tenido contacto sexual con una persona del sexo opuesto, corro todavía el riesgo de haber sido infectado(a)?

➤ Sí. El HIV no discrimina. Usted no tiene que ser un homosexual o una persona que se inyecta drogas para ser infectada.

➤ Tanto los hombres como las mujeres pueden ser infectados(as) y transmitir su infección a otra persona a través del contacto sexual.

➤ Si el compañero(a) sexual con quien tiene contacto ha tenido contacto sexual previo con alguien infectado(a), usted puede ser infectado(a).

¿Hay posibilidades de ser infectado con HIV al donar sangre?

➤ No. No hay ningún riesgo de contraer el HIV cuando usted dona sangre.

➤ Los centros de donación de sangre usan una aguja nueva y estéril para cada donación.

¿Puedo ser infectado(a) con HIV al usar el asiento de inodoro o por el uso de objetos de uso común?

➤ No. El HIV no vive en asientos de inodoro o en objetos de uso diario, aún en aquellos en que se pueden encontrar fluídos del cuerpo. Otros ejemplos de objetos de uso diario son tiradores de la puerta, teléfonos y fuentes de agua.

Una amiga me dijo que mientras estuviera tomando píldoras anticonceptivas, no corría riesgo de contraer el SIDA. ¿Es esto cierto?

➤ No. Las píldoras anticonceptivas no protegen a nadie contra el HIV.

➤ Usted puede ser infectada con HIV mientras usa píldoras anticonceptivas.

➤ La única manera segura de evitar la infección es: -evitar el compartir agujas. -abstenerse de relaciones sexuales, o tener estas sólo con una compañero que no esté infectado.

➤ Los condones de látex (aunque no están libres de peligro) se sabe que pueden prevenir la transmisión del HIV. Los condones se pueden romper durante el acto sexual. Uselos en forma apropiada cada vez que tenga contacto sexual de cualquier tipo.

➤ Aún si está tomando la píldora, usted puede usar un condón si tiene planes de tener contacto sexual con alguna persona que usted no está segura si está infectada o no.

¿Qué debo hacer si tengo sospechas de que he sido infectado(a) con HIV?

➤ Hable con alguna persona sobre la posibilidad de hacerse una prueba de HIV para determinar si está infectado(a). Esta persona puede ser uno de los padres, un médico, un trabajador(a) en el área de la salud o alguna persona que trabaje en un centro de consejo y diagnóstico de SIDA.

➤ Llame a la Línea telefónica de SIDA (1-800-342-AIDS) para saber a dónde ir para recibir consejo acerca de la prueba de HIV. No tiene que dar su nombre y su llamada es gratuita. Puede llamar también al departamento de salud del estado o local. El número aparece bajo Departamento de Salud en la sección de Gobierno de su guía telefónica.

➤ Su médico puede aconsejarle que reciba consejo y que reciba la prueba de SIDA si usted es hemofílico o si ha recibido transfusiones de sangre entre 1978 y 1985.

(La información fue provista por el centro para control de enfermedades con la excepción de las estadísticas de Nashville CARES)

Printed Resources for Help and Information

Johnson, Earvin "Magic", **What You Can Do to Avoid AIDS,** Time Books, a division of Random House, Inc. New York, © 1992 by Earvin "Magic" Johnson.

FREE FROM THE *DEPARTMENT OF HEALTH AND HUMAN SERVICES, PUBLIC HEALTH SERVICE, CENTERS FOR DISEASE CONTROL*

AIDS Prevention Guide For Parents And Other Adults Concerned About Youth. Contains fact sheets on: What Is HIV Infection? And What is AIDS?; How You Can And Cannot Become Infected With HIV; Common Questions, Accurate Answers; Talking With Young People About HIV Infection And AIDS; Deciding What To Say To Younger Children (Late Elementary And Middle School Aged)

Deciding What To Say To Teenagers (Junior And Senior High School Aged). Contains Handouts For Young People on: Information For Young People (Late Elementary And Middle School Aged); Information For Young People (Junior and Senior High School Aged); How To Join The Community Response; Where To Go For Further Information and Assistance.

Surgeon General's Report on Acquired Immune Deficiency Syndrome; pamphlet; contains more detailed information than the brochure.

HIV Infection And AIDS: Are You At Risk?

Preventing HIV & AIDS; HIV/NAIEP/1-92/013.

What About AIDS Testing?; U.S. Government Printing Office: 1988/535-727

Voluntary HIV Counseling and Testing: Facts, Issues, and Answers; NAIEP 9/91 D545

Caring For Someone With AIDS: Information For Friends, Relatives, Household Members, And Others Who Care For A Person With AIDS At Home

FROM CHANNING L. BETE CO., INC., SOUTH DEERFIELD, MA. 01373, ORDER PHONE 800-628-7733 (SCRIPTOGRAPHIC BOOKLETS)

A Christian Response to AIDS, © 1990, booklet number 46300.

What *Everyone* Should Know About AIDS (1992 edition) © 1983, booklet number 14274.

About Living With HIV (1991 edition) © 1990, booklet number 37689.

Making Responsible Choices About Sex (1991 edition) © 1987, booklet number 18788.

What Every Teenager Should Know About Peer Pressure (1991 edition) © 1987, booklet number 18820.

FROM HEALTH AND WELFARE MINISTRIES PROGRAM DEPARTMENT OF THE GENERAL BOARD OF GLOBAL MINISTRIES OF THE UNITED METHODIST CHURCH.

Worship Resource for HIV & AIDS Ministries by Patricia D. Brown and Adele K. Wilcox, Companion piece to the worship resource.

Enabling AIDS Ministries, pamphlet number 5088.

FROM AMERICAN SOCIAL HEALTH ASSOCIATION (A NATIONAL NONPROFIT ORGANIZATION DEDICATED TO THE ELIMINATION OF ALL STD'S). P.O. BOX 13827, RESEARCH TRIANGLE PARK, NC 27709, (919) 361-8400.

HIV Negative: When are you free from HIV? Information on testing and HIV prevention. Note: 900 number on the brochure should read 900-**230**-AIDS (900-230-2437).

Positive Living; a pamphlet for persons who have been diagnosed as HIV positive. The three parts of the booklet explain HIV infection and how to live with it, providing information on medical data and care, protecting yourself and others, and building support.

FROM THE AMERICAN RED CROSS (BROCHURES)

HIV Infection and AIDS
Testing for HIV Infection
Living With HIV Infection
Drugs, Sex, and AIDS
Children, Parents and AIDS
Teenagers and AIDS
Women, Sex, and AIDS
Men, Sex, and AIDS
School Systems and AIDS—Information for Teachers and School Officials
Your Job and AIDS: Are There Risks?
A Guide to Home Care for the Person With AIDS
HIV Infection and Workers in Health Care Settings

Recursos en español

DE LA CRUZ ROJA

La Infección por HIV y el SIDA (folleto)

Programa de prevención del SIDA en el lugar de trabajo

Programa de prevención del SIDA para adolescentes

Guía para Padres de Familias

Video ganador de un premio: "Beyond Fear"

¿Quién Será? (un libro de historietas)

Mi Hermano (fotonovela; también en inglés)

Video: **Mi Hermano**

DEL DEPARTMENTO DE SALUD Y SERVICIOS HUMANOS, SERVICIO DE SALUD PUBLICA, CENTROS PARA CONTROL DE ENFERMEDADES

Cuidando de alguien con SIDA: Información para amigos, familiares, personas que conviven y otras que cuidan de una persona con SIDA en el hogar

Informe del Jefe del Servicio de Salud Pública de los Estados Unidos sobre el Síndrome de Inmuno-Deficiencia Adquirida (AIDS)

Infección por HIV y SIDA: ¿Corre usted riesgo?

OTRAS

AIDS y las Drogas Intravenosas (Estado de Connecticut, Departamento de Salud Pública, Calle Washington 150, Hartford CT 06106)

SIDA O AIDS: Piénselo (Bridgeport Public Health Department)

Cuando un Amigo Tiene AIDS (Gay Men's Health Crisis)

Las Mujeres y el SIDA (Impact AIDS, Inc., 3692 18th Street, San Francisco, CA 94110)

Lo Que *TODOS* Deben Saber Sobre el SIDA (folleto numero 14308). From Channing L. Bete Co., Inc., South Deerfield, MA. 01373, Order phone (800) 628-7733 (Scriptographic Booklets)

Where to Go for Help

ORGANIZATIONS

American Social Health Association (ASHA) P.O. Box 13827, Research Triangle Park, NC 27709, (919) 361-8400.

CDC National AIDS Hotline: confidential and anonymous information on HIV and AIDS, referral to local health care organizations, counselors, and support groups

English: (800) 342-2437 (always open)
Spanish: (800) 344-7432 (8:00 A.M.-2:00 A.M. eastern time, Monday-Friday)
TTY/TDD (800) 243-7889 (10:00 A.M.-10:00 P.M. eastern time, Monday-Friday)

CDC National STD Hotline: confidential and anonymous information on all sexually transmitted diseases, referral for health care and support groups
(800) 227-8922, (8:00 A.M.-11:00 P.M. eastern time, Monday-Friday)

AIDS Clinical Trials Information Service (ACTIS): Information on new drug trials for HIV and AIDS that are sponsored by the government. 9:00 A.M.-7:00 P.M. Eastern time, Monday-Friday

English and Spanish: (800) 874-2572
TTY/TDD (800) 243-7012

Project Inform: information on clinical drug treatments

People With AIDS Coalition: self-empowerment information for people with HIV and AIDS 10:00 A.M.-6:00 P.M. eastern time, Monday-Friday (800) 828-3280

HIV Nightline: Crisis calls and emotional support for people with HIV 12:00 A.M.-8:00 A.M. Monday-Friday, 8:00 P.M.-8:00 A.M. Saturday and Sunday (415) 668-2437 (800-273-2437 in N. CA only)

CDC National AIDS Clearinghouse: educational materials on HIV and AIDS, P.O. Box 6003, Rockville, MD 20849-6003 (800) 458-5231

American Medical Association, Task Force on AIDS, 535 North Dearborn, Chicago, IL 60610, (312) 464-4566

American Red Cross, AIDS Education Office, 1709 New York Avenue NW, Suite 208, Washington, D.C. 20006, (202) 639-3223

National Council of Churches/AIDS Task Force, 475 Riverside Drive, Room 572, New York, NY 10115, (212) 870-2421

The Pediatric AIDS Foundation (213) 395-9051

RACIAL/ETHNIC/CULTURAL ORGANIZATIONS
American Indian Health Care Association (612) 293-0233

Association of Asian/Pacific Community Health Organizations (510) 272-9536

Bienestar: Gay and Lesbian Latinos Unidos (213) 660-9680

Blacks Educating Blacks About Sexual Health Issues (BEBASHI) (215) 546-4140

Coalition of Hispanic and Human Services Organizations (COSSMHO) (202) 387-5000

Gay Men's Health Crisis—AIDS Hotline (212) 807-6655

Girl's, Inc. (212) 689-3700

National Gay and Lesbian Task Force (202) 332-6483

National Minority AIDS Council (800) 669-5052

National Native American AIDS Prevention Center (800) 283-AIDS

SERVICES FOR TEENS
The National Youth Crisis Hotline (800) 448-4663

AIDS Hotline for Teens (staffed by trained high school students) (800) 234-TEEN

IYG Gay/Lesbian Youth Hotline (800) 347-TEEN

National Network of Runaway and Youth Services (202) 682-4114

The National Runaway Switchboard (24 hour hotline) (800) 621-4000

The National Youth Crisis Hotline (800) 448-4663